Cleft Palate and Associated Speech Characteristics

by

RAYMOND MASSENGILL, Jr.
Assistant Dean and Director
of Medical Education
East Tennessee State University

and

PHYLLIS P. PHILLIPS
Speech and Hearing Clinic
Auburn University

CLIFFS NOTES, INC. · LINCOLN, NEBRASKA

Library of Congress Catalog Card No.: 73–89776
ISBN   0–8220–1801–2
© Copyright 1975 by Cliffs Notes, Inc.

Contents

Chapter 1

Fundamentals of Congenital Clefts of the Lip and Palate

Introduction

During the past century, and certainly during the past decade, a better understanding of cleft palate and associated speech characteristics has been formulated, but there are still a number of unanswered questions. Modern research by the members of the cleft-palate team—which includes speech pathologists and speech scientists, plastic, maxillofacial, and oral surgeons, and various dental specialists, otolaryngologists, audiologists, psychologists, pediatricians, social workers, and others—has changed many of the old beliefs and treatment procedures. Moreover, objective research findings have presented new questions that must also be explored.

The "Authors' Guide" for Cliffs Speech and Hearing Series indicates that the overview treatment provided in this series of publications is intended to "prepare the reader, particularly the beginning student, for a more thorough investigation of the area through numerous other materials and resources" (1). The present authors endorse this goal and have attempted to fulfill it in this book. In addition, it is their hope that lay people, and most especially parents of cleft-palate children, will be helped to gain a better understanding of the problem. The Glossary at the end of this book will enable lay readers and beginning students to develop a familiarity with the technical terms used by the professionals who make up the cleft-palate team.

Since this book offers only an overview of cleft palate and associated speech characteristics, the authors recommend that the reader continue the study and exploration of this complex subject through the use of more detailed and more specialized materials and resources.

Incidence of Cleft Palate

Studies too numerous to mention have been conducted regarding the incidence of congenital cleft lip/palate. The conclusions of these investigations have not all been in complete agreement. The incidence, as reported by Pickrell in 1971, is basic for the present book. He stated:

7

General information regarding cleft of the lip [is as follows]: The incidence is approximately 1 in 700 births. It occurs more commonly in boys than in girls, the ratio being about 60 to 40 and because of reasons that remain very very obscure seemingly the left side is affected a little bit more frequently than the right side. Now 25% of these patients will have only a cleft of the lip. Seventy-five percent of the patients with the cleft of the lip will also have an associated cleft of the palate. But an additional 25% will have only a cleft of the palate without an associated cleft of the lip so that you see either cleft of the lip or cleft of the palate may occur independently although 75% of the patients with cleft of the lip will also have an associated cleft of the palate (2).

Fogh-Anderson points out that "of all congenital deformities, cleft lip and palate have for years been considered as belonging to the most common. They seem to occur among all peoples of the earth, and have been known [since] before the time of Christ" (3).

Considering the high incidence of cleft palate, it is highly likely that most speech-pathologists will have an opportunity during their careers to work with some of these patients. Likewise, most people will at some time be associated with persons having a cleft of the palate. A familiarity with the problem will provide the foundation for relationships based on understanding and knowledge rather than on lack of knowledge, hearsay, and superstition.

Etiology

Olin states that Arey's theory indicates that "clefts of the lip and palate are developmental deformities which result when one or more of the embryonic processes of the face fail to fuse or unite with the adjacent processes during the first trimester of pregnancy" (4).

There appears to be no one definite cause for this developmental deformity. Zemlin writes that "intrauterine anoxia, toxic poisoning, high concentrations of cortisone, and heredity seem to be related to cleft palate. After an exhaustive study of etiological factors, Fogh-Anderson in Denmark, concluded that heredity is in all likelihood the most essential factor for cleft palate and cleft lip" (5).

Lane (6) discusses drugs that are known to induce cleft lip or cleft palate in experimental animals, and Longacre also elaborates on this factor. Longacre points to the work of Warkany (7), who produced "cleft palates in rats by riboflavin lack." He writes that Deuschle, Geiger, and Warkany (8) "produced cleft palates with hypervitaminosis," and that Fraser, Fainstat, and Kalter (9) ' produced cleft palates in mice by injection of cortisone during the organogenetic phase." He also states that "Warkany [10] reported the birth of a malformed child with partial cleft palate following an unmarried mother taking aninopterin as an abortifacient" (11). The thalidomide tragedy was mentioned also by Longacre (11) as well as by Lane (6).

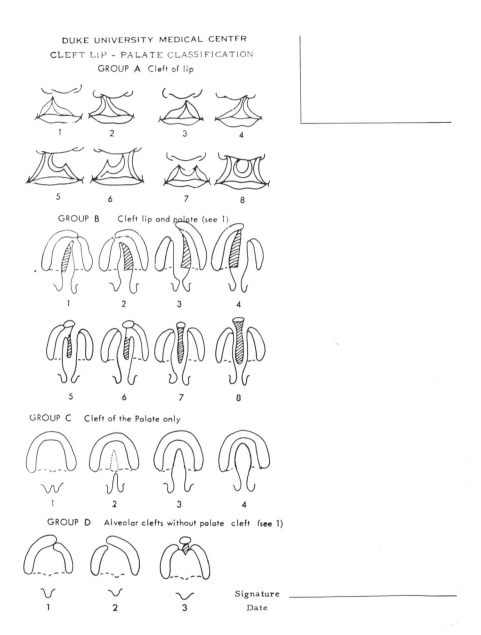

Fig. 1.1. Duke University Medical Center cleft lip-cleft palate statistical and clinical history card

Congenital clefts have been known to be present in calves, monkeys, dogs, and other animals. Many times these animals die shortly after birth because of inability to nurse properly and because the owners are not familiar with the correct methods of caring for the deformed animals. It has been the authors' experience, in talking with some of the owners of animals that have produced offspring with clefts, that the owners wanted to get rid of the offspring and the parent as soon as possible so that others would not think their breeding stock was producing deviate or abnormal animals. As a partial result of this philosophy, cleft-palate animals have been difficult to locate. Once they are located it is expensive to raise such animals because of the special care and attention they need when they are young. The senior author has one adult boxer dog with an open cleft lip and palate, and it is cared for like any other ordinary dog, but this dog was obtained after he was full-grown.

Classification

There are numerous types of clefts, including clefts of the lip, clefts of the palate, and clefts of the lip and palate. There are clefts so small that they involve only a fraction of the soft palate, and clefts so large as to constitute a complete cleft of the soft palate, hard palate, alveolar ridge, and both sides of the lip. The smallest and least significant of the anatomical conditions associated with cleft lip/palate is the bifid uvula. This is simply a small division, or split, in the middle of the uvula, the small portion of the soft palate, which can be observed hanging at the back of the soft palate. Although this is technically a palatal cleft of the smallest degree, it usually receives little attention; therefore, it is not a consideration in this book.

Any classification system represents an effort to construct a system that will communicate descriptions of patients, lend itself to enhancing an understanding of the relationship among parts, and serve both student and researcher in study and investigation. Different methods of classification have been employed to describe the various types of clefting conditions. Figure 1.1 shows the Duke University Medical Center Cleft Lip–Cleft Palate Statistical and Clinical History Card.*

As already indicated, there are many types of clefts and combinations of clefts. One of the simplest and most widely used classification systems is that of Veau. Figure 1.2 illustrates the Veau classifications, which are as follows:

A. Veau I—soft palate cleft only.

B. Veau II—soft palate and hard palate cleft.

C. Veau III—soft palate and hard palate cleft but with a unilateral cleft extending into the upper alveolar ridge and upper lip.

* Permission to use this card was obtained from Dr. Kenneth Pickrell, Chairman and Professor of the Division of Plastic and Maxillofacial Surgery, Duke University Medical Center.

D. Veau IV—soft palate and hard palate cleft but with a bilateral cleft in the upper alveolar ridge and upper lip (12).

More complicated and involved classification systems, although having merit in their completeness, have the disadvantage of being so complicated that they discourage use.

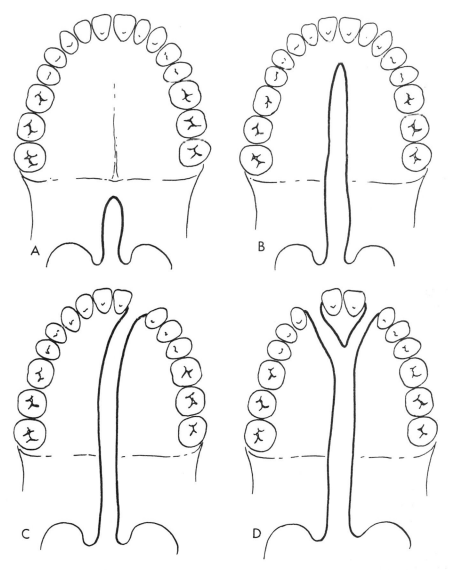

Fig. 1.2. Veau's categorization of clefts: *A*, Veau I; *B*, Veau II; *C*, Veau III; *D*, Veau IV

Chapter 2

Counseling with the Family of the Cleft Lip/Palate Child

The Cleft-Palate Team as Counselors

The cleft can be as limited as that shown in Figure 2.1 (Veau I), which is a cleft of the soft palate only, or as severe as that shown in Figure 2.2 (Veau IV), which is a bilateral cleft of the lip and a complete cleft of the palate. There also can be a cleft of the soft palate and hard palate, as shown in Figure 2.3 (Veau II), and there are a number of other combinations, as indicated in Chapter 1.

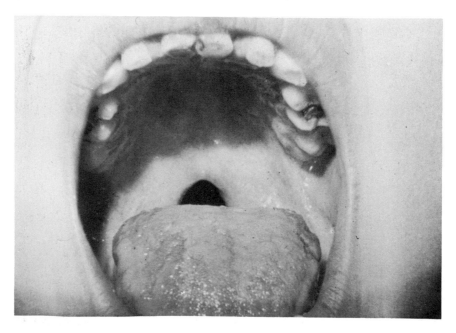

Fig. 2.1. Cleft of soft palate only (Veau I)

12

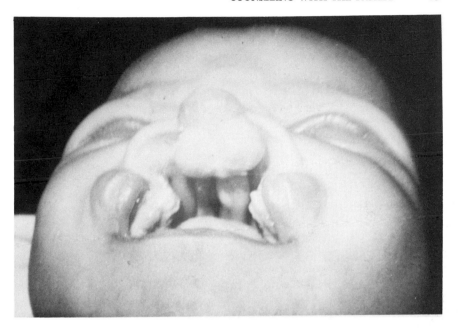

Fig. 2.2. Floating type premaxilla, bilateral cleft of lip and palate (Veau IV)

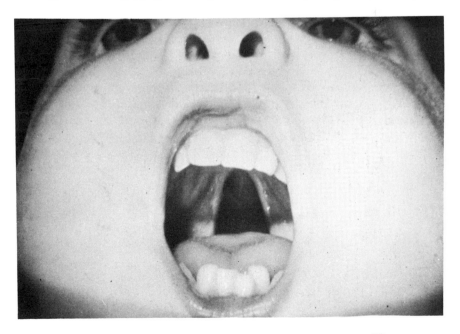

Fig. 2.3. Cleft of the soft palate and hard palate only (Veau II)

The authors have found the utilization of pictures to be a successful technique in dealing with the family of a cleft-palate child. Figures 2.4–2.9 are a case presentation following one patient from shortly after birth through most of his surgery. The patient was born with a left complete cleft lip and palate. Figure 2.4 shows the patient at the age of approximately nine weeks. Figure 2.5 shows the same patient at approximately eleven weeks of age after the lip had been surgically closed. Figure 2.6 shows the patient at the age of approximately four months, Figure 2.7 at approximately eighteen months, Figure 2.8 at approximately two years, and Figure 2.9 at approximately twelve years of age. Obviously these pictures represent a long and rather complicated rehabilitation program involving much teamwork and long-range planning.

By the use of pictures, as just reviewed, the specialists on the cleft-palate team can show the parents of the cleft lip/palate child what can be accomplished. Careful study of this case presentation will readily enable the reader to appreciate the number of specialists who may be needed to care for such a child during his rehabilitation.

The Cleft-Palate Team

The cleft-palate team consists of the obstetrician, pediatrician, plastic surgeon, orthodontist and prosthodontist, speech pathologist, psychologist, social worker, otolaryngologist, and audiologist. We should also consider the parents as members of the cleft-palate team, for much of the speech teaching, and the responsibility of keeping appointments, following the directions of the specialists, and reporting, can best be done by informed, cooperative parents. The following is a description of the role of each member of the cleft-palate team.

Obstetrician

The obstetrician is usually the first specialist to observe the cleft lip/palate baby. He may choose to tell the parents of the cleft condition alone or with other members of the cleft-palate team. The importance of what can be done for the cleft-palate child must be fully explained to the parents. Often members of the cleft-palate team try to see the baby and his parents professionally as soon after birth as possible.

"Breaking the news" to the family is usually done within twenty-four hours after the birth of the child; it is generally felt that the job is the attending physician's responsibility. Not all parents are counseled about the baby's

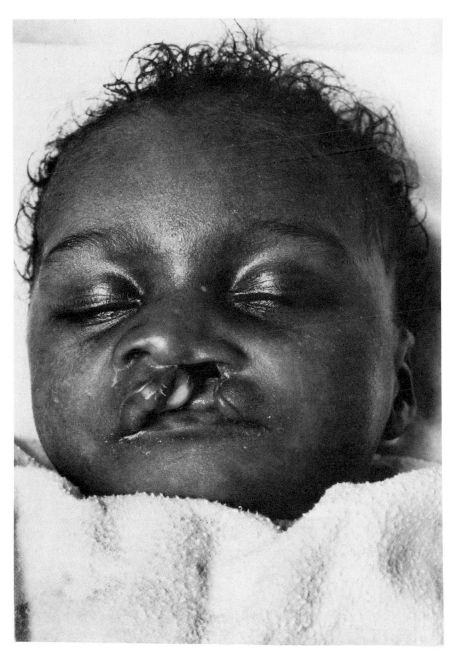

Fig. 2.4. Patient with a left complete cleft lip and palate at the age of approximately nine weeks

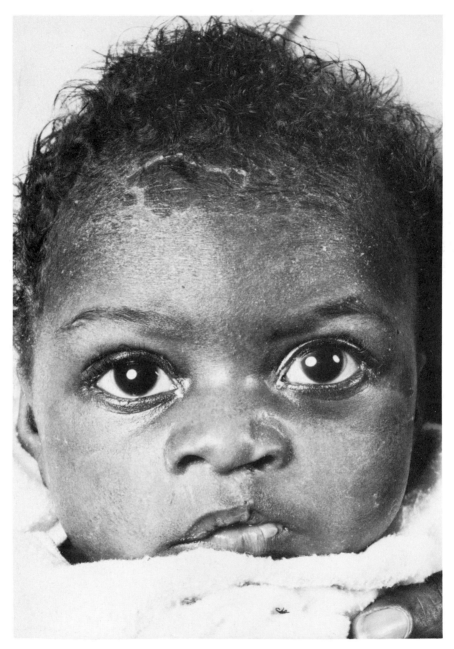

Fig. 2.5. Patient at age of approximately eleven weeks after the lip had been surgically closed

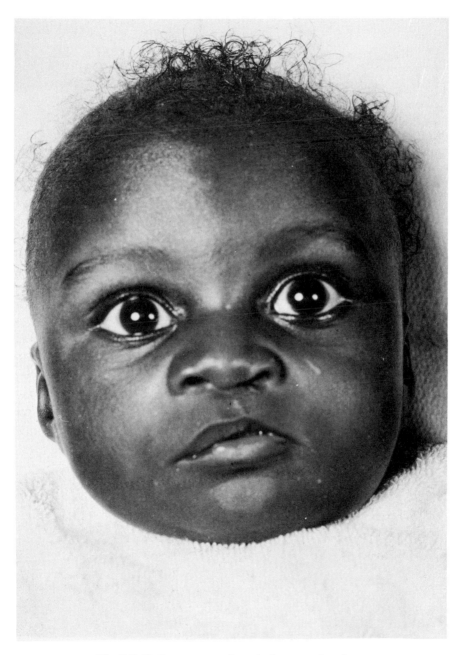

Fig. 2.6. Patient at approximately four months of age

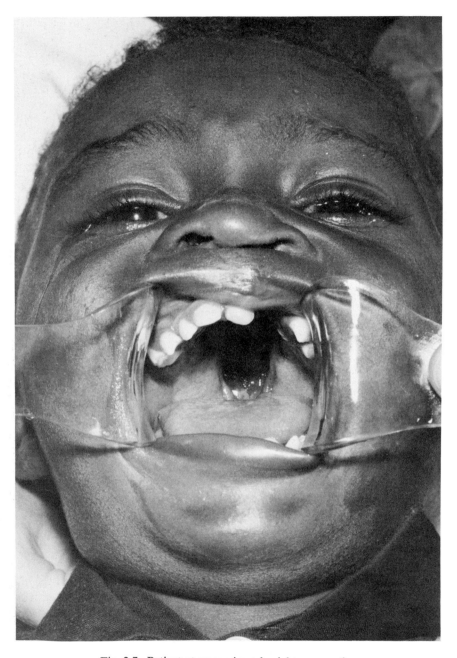

Fig. 2.7. Patient at approximately eighteen months

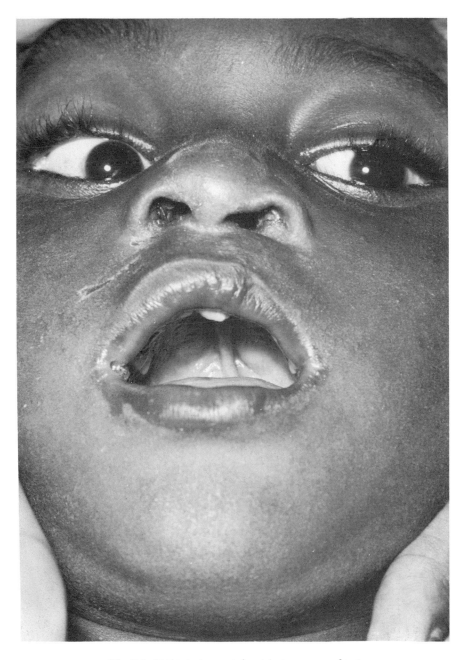

Fig. 2.8. Patient at approximately two years of age

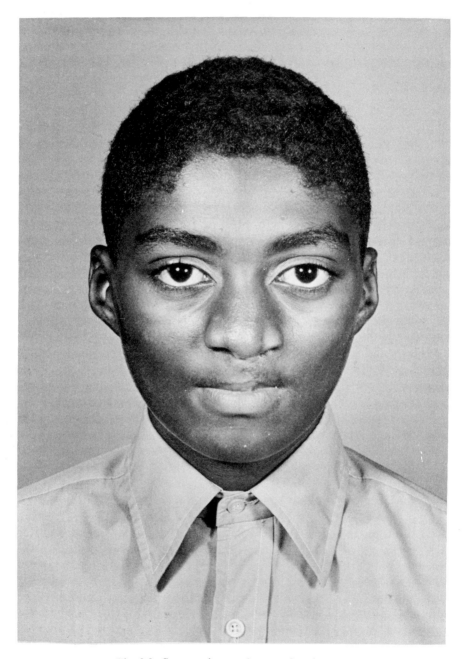

Fig. 2.9. Same patient at the age of twelve years

condition immediately following delivery. Sometimes this is because of the emotional state of one or both parents at the time of the birth of the baby or because of other physical anomalies of the child. Also, not all clefts are discovered immediately following delivery. The cleft lip is all too apparent and can scarcely escape the attention of any observer, but the palate is not so readily observable. Therefore, clefts that are confined to the palate may not be detected without adequate postnatal examination. Even with specific examination some small clefts may be overlooked until the child grows in size, with concomitant growth in the size of the palatal opening and resultant associated problems.

Pediatrician

The pediatrician is usually the next specialist to see the baby after the obstetrician. He will check the baby from a pediatric standpoint and will usually refer the patient to other members of the cleft-palate team. The pediatric nurse will advise the mother about different aspects of nursing as applied to the cleft lip/palate child. Such matters as proper position during nursing and proper bottle nipple most advantageous for the young baby will be reviewed by this specialist. The booklet by Snyder, Berkowitz, Bozch, and Stool, *Your Cleft Lip and Palate Child: A Basic Guide for Parents* (13), provides most useful information concerning feeding procedures.

The pediatrician is in charge of the general health of the baby, but he will often counsel the parents concerning many aspects of the child's growth and development. The usual concerns of parents of new babies are shared by the parents of cleft-palate children, but there are certain special concerns.

Feeding. This, of course, is of immediate concern for the health of the infant. Because of the mouth deformity, feeding presents a special problem. The immediacy of this concern gives feeding a high-priority rating in the parent counseling provided by the pediatrician.

Surgical repair. Another high-priority subject in the parent counseling is a description of surgical-repair plans for the infant. Although the pediatrician does not perform surgical repair, he is often the person who initiates the informational conferences with the parents and contacts the plastic surgeon.

Plastic Surgeon

The plastic surgeon is often the chairman of the cleft-palate team. After the pediatrician refers the child to the cleft-palate team, the plastic surgeon will be the first one to examine the child. It is his responsibility to explain to the parents the actual surgical procedures that may be utilized to correct the deformity. The importance of the child being in the hands of a highly specialized plastic surgeon cannot be overemphasized. The following quotation from a publication by such specialists well illustrates this point:

> It has often been said of cleft lip that there is no group of cases in which good results are more important or in which bad results show so plainly. The child's life, future, health, welfare, and happiness are at stake when the decision is made to repair the lip (14).

Although plastic surgery is commonly thought of as being a modern specialization, and rightfully so in its present form, it has a long and complicated history. The recorded accounts of attempts to close cleft palates surgically disclose some rather unbelievable procedures. These accounts might be interesting for general readers and are certainly academically pertinent to the speech pathologist's reading, but they would serve little purpose here other than pointing out the historical development of cleft-palate surgery.

The surgical procedures available today, however, are pertinent to the discussion that the plastic surgeon will have with the parents. There is no one preferred surgical procedure since each cleft is different, each cleft-palate child has a different face, and growth patterns differ from one individual to another. Adequate counseling from the plastic surgeon will do much to aid the parents in understanding a number of important aspects of their child's care, including:

1. The need for surgery.
2. What is involved in the actual surgery.
3. The reasons why one child may be treated with one method and another child with a different procedure.
4. The responsibility that parents have in keeping appointments and complying with care instructions.

It must be remembered that parents with similar problems discuss these problems with each other. Without an adequate understanding of treatment procedures confusion may arise. For instance, when one parent tells another parent about a surgical procedure employed with a given child, the second parent may generalize that his child should have been treated in the same manner.

The significance of adequate parent counseling concerning plastic surgery cannot be underestimated; but this is only a part of the plastic surgeon's work. His work with the child also involves such things as examination of the cleft, deciding on the appropriate procedures to be employed, following the growth patterns of the child's face, effecting the repair in the indicated steps, and evaluating the effectiveness of the work done. After the plastic surgeon has completed his initial examination of the child and counseled with the parents, the next specialists to be seen are those in dentistry.

Orthodontist

The cleft lip/palate child will need regular dental care and should be seen by a dentist routinely. This is not merely the normal dental care recommended for all children. The cleft-palate child has more dental problems than the normal child, and at the same time he has a greater need than the normal child for properly aligned and healthy teeth. Teeth must be preserved since prosthetic and orthodontic devices, if used, must be attached to the teeth. Furthermore, a mouth with a cleft presents special difficulty in the use of false teeth since dentures will not stay firm in the mouth, thus increasing the necessity of maintaining optimum dental health. This need is complicated by the fact that dental malformations are the rule rather than the exception in cleft-palate children. Since the mouth structures are malaligned and deformed, teeth may be rotated, deformed, tilted, incompletely erupted, or malpositioned. Some teeth may be missing since the buds from which they should have developed may never have formed. In other cases there may be too many teeth. In other words, the distortion of relationships of structures results in some unusual dental arrangements.

In addition, the dentist or orthodontist is faced with some nonmedical problems. Perhaps the most common is the feeling on the part of the parents that, since the teeth are in such bad condition already, they are hardly worth the money and effort to care for them. The old feeling that really poor teeth might as well be allowed to decay and fall out must be combated by the orthodontist in his educational program with both the parents and the child. A second nonmedical problem faced by the orthodontist involves the child's preconditioning to face further oral repair. The child has already sustained sufficient oral insult to cause reluctance to seek more. Dental specialists, then, must be able to convince both parents and patient of the importance of dental care.

The cleft lip/palate child should be seen by the dentist at least by the age of three years. The following three stages of the orthodontic program are often needed during cleft-palate rehabilitation after the deciduous dentition (baby teeth) has developed:

1. Expansion of the maxillary segment around the age of three or four.
2. Incisor and molar correction at the age of six or seven.
3. Cuspid and bicuspid treatment after permanent teeth eruption (4).

In programs calling for bone grafting, a most specialized technique, the orthodontist may work closely with the plastic surgeon. Appliances like the one shown in Figure 2.10 are sometimes used by the orthodontist to help promote a better palatal arch. The orthodontist has at his disposal other such appliances for use in the cleft-palate habilitation program. Such appliances

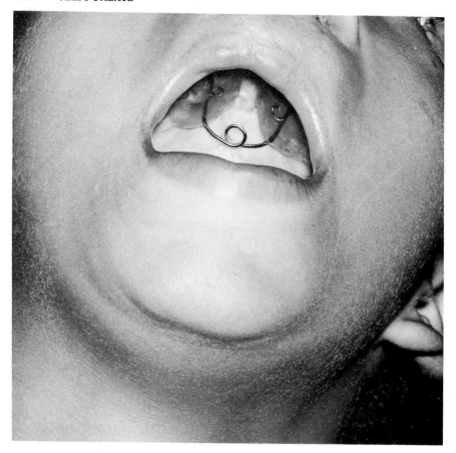

Fig. 2.10. Expansion appliance used in the orthodontic program to help promote a better palatal arch

are individually prescribed for each patient, and no two children will indicate identical treatment. Counseling with the parents may aid in their acceptance of the prescribed program and of their part in maintenance. Parents' acceptance and support of the dental program enhances the child's acceptance of the appliance and the necessary dental care.

Another specialist on the cleft-palate team is the prosthodontist, the maker of the prosthesis, or appliance, that may be needed by the child.

Speech Pathologist

The speech pathologist may see the child shortly after birth along with the plastic surgeon. The speech pathologist will explain to the parents the way speech and language develop normally—that is, when certain words should be produced and at what age the child should be saying words and phrases.

If the child has only a cleft of the lip and lip surgery is successful, then a speech problem is unlikely. But if there is a cleft of the alveolar ridge and the palate, two types of speech problem, nasality and poor articulation, may be present. Sometimes the parents of a cleft-palate child, having heard an individual who has had an unsuccessful repair speak, tend to feel that all cleft-palate children talk in that manner. They have heard the nasal speech and observed the twitching of the nasal grimace the child produces when talking. At this point it is most important for the speech pathologist to point out that not all cleft-palate children talk alike. He must explain the cause of the hypernasality in the child the parents have heard talking in an unsatisfactory manner, and he must tell them what the cleft-palate team is going to do to prevent this from happening with their child. The speech pathologist should explain in the simplest terms possible the role of the soft palate and the throat or pharyngeal wall during speech production and the ways they relate to nasality.

As Snyder, Berkowitz, Bzoch, and Stool have written:

A definite relationship exists between speech and the function of the soft palate. Muscles of the soft palate and the throat must work together to close off the back opening to the nose to make most speech sounds in the mouth (13).

Moreover, as Massengill has pointed out:

When the soft palate does not meet with the pharyngeal wall during speech, an opening between the soft palate and the throat is present, by which speech can escape into the nasal cavity and may be perceived as nasality (15).

Figure 2.11 shows the soft palate not meeting with the pharyngeal wall (throat) during speech—as a result of this condition, much of the speech

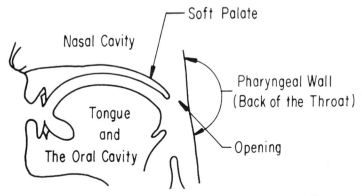

Fig. 2.11. Soft palate not meeting the pharyngeal wall

sound is coming out through the nose. Figure 2.12 shows the soft palate meeting with the back of the throat and helping to close off this opening so that the speech can be directed more through the mouth. Such diagrams may be extremely helpful to the speech pathologist in explaining to the parents the cause for the nasal sound in their child's speech; such diagrams are also helpful in directly explaining the same matters to older patients. An understanding of the anatomical basis for the nasality aids in preventing the feeling that the correction of nasality involves simply "trying harder," which in turn facilitates rehabilitation procedures.

The speech pathologist and the plastic surgeon will explain to the parents that the relationship where the soft palate meets with the pharyngeal wall during speech is the type of condition that will be strived for in surgery. Sometimes more than one surgical procedure may be necessary to obtain this velopharyngeal relationship.

The other speech problem that the child with a cleft of the alveolar ridge and palate may encounter is that of faulty articulation. Morley, in her discussion of faulty articulation, indicated that this problem may be present as a result of "inability to produce certain consonants, due to the anatomical deformity of the mouth" (16). This may result in one sound being substituted for another—for example, /t/ being substituted for /s/, as in *taw* for *saw*—or, if the teeth do not come together properly, in a lisp being produced during speech production. In the articulation-problem category, sounds may also be omitted from words and additional sounds may be added, thus increasing the chance of the word being misarticulated. Obviously, the combination of the two problems, nasality and articulation, results in speech that is disturbing to the listener because of both its distinctive sound and its loss of intelligibility.

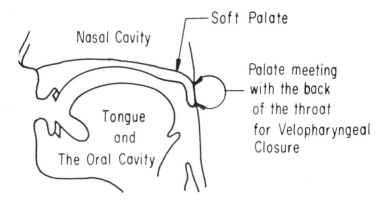

Fig. 2.12. Soft palate meeting with the pharyngeal wall for complete velopharyngeal closure

The speech pathologist is one of the key counselors for both the patient and his family from the time of the patient's birth for as long as the cleft-palate team continues to see the patient. More will be explained about different aspects of speech in the following chapter. A more detailed description of the varied aspects of the speech pathologist's role is found in the final chapter of this book.

Psychologist

The physicians on the cleft-palate team may call on a psychologist to see the parents of the child shortly after the child's birth. The psychologist will help them to cope with any negative reactions they are experiencing, and he will explain, along with the other members of the cleft-palate team, what can be done for the child. He will also deal with any questions the parents have concerning educational or psychological problems the child may encounter. Parents are usually concerned about how their child will function in society. His potential for learning speech, attending regular schools, and developing normal social relationships are all parental concerns that need consideration. Furthermore, parents may experience upsetting feelings concerning their child's deformity and may need counseling from the psychologist relative to their own feelings of guilt, hurt, and disappointment.

The psychologist will also be available to provide additional aid for the parents and the patient if it is needed as the child grows and develops. Obviously, the cleft-palate patient should be referred to a psychologist if he is maladjusted to the extent that his psychological problems interfere with his ability to seek corrective therapy and profit from it. The psychologist, too, will aid the speech pathologist in analyzing the patient's intellectual capacity.

Basically, the psychologist's responsibilities lie in two areas: (1) the problems of the parents and (2) the problems of the child. Since these responsibilities may be dealt with by specialists other than the psychologist—that is, the speech pathologist or the social worker—they will be discussed further along with other problems associated with cleft palate.

Social Worker

The social worker can aid the family and the patient in a number of diversified ways. If the patient's family is indigent, this specialist can help them contact the appropriate agency (such as the crippled children's section of the state board of health) for financial aid needed for the habilitation program. The social worker may also be called on by members of the cleft-palate team to make home visits, to see if certain programs are being carried out as previously instructed, or to obtain needed information. The social worker may also help arrange for transportation, lodging, and other needs when the family comes to the medical center or rehabilitation center.

The above duties are only a sampling of what the social worker may be called upon to perform. The speech pathologist relies on the social worker as his liaison person, for it is often the social worker who coordinates the habilitation program. This is particularly true when the family is not sufficiently able, whether because of indifference, lack of finances, or lack of education, to understand the scope of the problem sufficiently to follow through with the long habilitation program.

Otolaryngologist and Audiologist

Cleft-palate children have a higher incidence of ear infections and hearing losses than children without clefts. Although there are a number of variables affecting incidence figures, such as age of child, type of cleft, degree of cleft, intelligence of child, type of physical management of the cleft, and so forth, the incidence of hearing pathology is clearly greater among cleft-palate children. The type of hearing loss exhibited is usually bilateral and conductive. Several factors may be involved in the cause of the hearing problems, but basically it can be assumed that the abnormal structures contribute to an abnormal relationship of structures. Obviously, the opening between the oral and nasal cavities allows for an abnormal articulation of these areas. Furthermore, the Eustachian-tube function may be influenced by the abnormal insertion of the muscles involved or by surgical procedures that have altered these functions.

Another concern of the otolaryngologist is the careful attention given to maintaining adenoidal tissue as an added aid in effecting closure where there is insufficient tissue otherwise. Careful attention to the possible function of adenoidal tissue should be given to all children because of the possible need for these tissues in the case of children with a submucous cleft. This is a condition in which the muscular tissues of the soft palate, and sometimes the bone of the hard palate, are cleft, but the covering of mucous membrane is intact.

Audiological assessment is of obvious importance to a population in which there is an unusually high incidence of hearing problems, in which there are speech and language problems, and in which speech therapy is to be expected. It is imperative that the speech pathologist know the child's hearing acuity and that the child's hearing health be maintained during the period of therapy.

As a part of providing the particular services needed in these two areas, the otolaryngologist and the audiologist may also counsel with the family and patient concerning different aspects of otolaryngology and audiology as they relate to the cleft-palate habilitation program.

Chapter 3

Speech

Van Riper has indicated that no one can work in the speech-therapy field for very long "without being confronted by the odd honking snort of cleft-palate speech" (17). McDonald has pointed out that when parents of cleft-palate children were asked what they "worried about more than anything else," most frequently they replied that they were worried about "how their children will talk" (18).

After the speech pathologist has established rapport with the family of the cleft-palate child, he should explain certain aspects of normal speech and language development. He may want to point out when the first words are usually said and when two- or three-word phrases are usually uttered.

Morley states that "speech is usually not established at the earliest until towards the end of the second year of life, but the actual sounds used in speech are acquired very much earlier" (16). Speech is learned, and for the most part the child will learn to speak from his parents or those most closely associated with him. "Normal children start imitating the sounds of adults in the second six months and rapidly get better at it" (19). This is one of the primary reasons why early counseling by the speech pathologist with the parents of the cleft-palate child is so important.

The parents should encourage the child from birth on to produce sounds and use his voice. Parents should start reading and singing to the baby very early in the child's life. Bzoch has indicated that "by one year of age children love vocal games," such as pat-a-cake, and that "repeating parts of rhymes" and "'talking' without real words can be fun for both mother and child" (13). Hahn has indicated that when the child is ten to fifteen months of age his parents will engage him in naming "all objects he touches or looks at," and will "invite imitation of words beginning with /p/, /b/, /m/, /w/, /t/, /d/, /n/, /l/, and even /r/" (20). Since the palate may not be closed at this early age, the parents should be taught "to settle for near accuracy in the placement of the articulators" (20) of the speech mechanism, such as the tongue and lips, when listening to their child talk. Hahn goes on to indicate that "after the palate is closed, /k/ and /g/ can be added to the repertoire" (20).

First words should be encouraged when the child is one year old and short sentences at two years (16). "At approximately 3 years of age the child may be producing 4 word sentences. Around 4 years of age the child may be talking in sentences which his parents and friends may easily understand" (21).

A method the senior author has used with parents of cleft-palate children is to have them keep a list of sounds and words the child produces and the date thereof. By this method, along with observation of the child, the speech pathologist can obtain a fairly accurate account of how well speech and language are developing at an early age. If a language deficit is expected, then detailed language testing will be attempted.

Parents often want to know when their child is likely to acquire certain sounds. The following list of the ages at which specific consonant sounds are usually obtained may be useful: /m/, /n/, /ng/, /p/, /f/, /h/, at age three; /y/ at age three and one-half; /k/, /b/, /d/, /g/, /r/ at age four; /s/, /sh/, /ch/ at age five; /t/, /voiceless th/, /v/, /l/, at age six; /voiced th/, /z/, /zh/, /j/ at age seven (22). As Georgiade, Clifford, and Massengill have commented:

> The importance of reading to the child and talking with the child every day from birth on cannot be overemphasized. Phonetic books and phonetic games written and produced according to the age level of the child are most useful in relationship to speech and language acquisition. These phonetic books and games can be found in many department or book stores (21).

Speech Problems Encountered by the Cleft-Palate Individual

The two major speech problems encountered by the cleft-palate child are hypernasality and poor articulation. In her discussion dealing with the assessment of speech, Morley states:

> Observations should include tests for the degree of nasopharyngeal occlusion, the development of language, and the use of articulation as language develops. Advice to the mother may be useful at any time, but, if surgery has been successful, speech therapy may be postponed until the child is at least four years of age, and then only if adequate progress is not occurring spontaneously (16).

Aspects of speech and language development and testing have already been discussed; the remainder of this chapter will deal with nasality and the articulation problems often encountered by the cleft-palate child.

Nasality

"Hypernasality has often had a different meaning for each of the specialists concerned with its cause and treatment. What may be heard as hypernasal voice quality by one individual may not be so heard by another" (15). Hypernasality is a complex phenomenon, and the senior author has devoted an entire book (15) to considerations concerning the subject. In the present book, however, since it is designed primarily for the beginning student and the lay reader, certain basic working definitions are employed.

Nasality is the quality of speech sounds when the nasal cavity is used as a resonator, especially when there is too much nasal resonance (23).

Nasal emission is the escape of air through the nose preventing normal production of most consonant sounds due to deficit or malfunction of the soft palate (23).

A student in the area of speech pathology will be confronted with the two above terms when he reviews the literature in the cleft-palate field as well as when he attends conferences, symposiums, and meetings on cleft-palate habilitation and, of course, during his clinical work. Other terms, such as *nasopharyngeal occlusion, palatopharyngeal closure, velopharyngeal closure,* and *velopharyngeal seal* or *velopharyngeal sufficiency,* relate to the soft palate or velum meeting with the pharyngeal wall during speech production. As explained in Chapter 2, "when the soft palate does not meet with the pharyngeal wall during speech, an opening between the soft palate and the throat is present, by which speech can escape into the nasal cavity and may be perceived as nasality" (15).

Evaluation Procedures

The cleft-palate child will be followed routinely by the speech pathologist from birth on. Around the age of three and one-half or four years it may be necessary to conduct specific testing procedures in regard to possible nasality. It is expected that the palate has been closed by this age.

Listening Test concerning Voice Quality. A rating scale concerning the degree of nasality is sometimes employed. Often this is a 5-point scale with zero meaning normal resonance and 5 meaning severe hypernasality. Westlake and Rutherford have written: "The vowels /i/ and /u/ between plosive and fricative consonants reveal nasality well. Words like *peep* and *shoes,* and phrases like *She likes high boots* are useful tests" (19). They indicate that the patient also should be listened to during conversation and oral reading to help "determine how altering pitch, rate, and intensity affect nasality" (19).

The speech clinician may also obtain some indication of the presence or absence of nasality when he is conducting the articulation examination. The latter part of this chapter will deal with articulation.

Intraoral Air-Pressure Testing. Numerous techniques and procedures have been used for intraoral air-pressure testing. Among these are the following:

1. "Ability to blow through the mouth without nasal escape of air" (16).
2. A gauged instrument like a manometer can be used to help determine the amount of oral air pressure the patient can produce with and without the nostrils occluded. "If the speaker is able to impound more air pressure while the nostrils are occluded, the examiner will assume that there is some leakage through the velopharyngeal valve" (4). The article by Morris concerning the use of the oral manometer as a diagnostic tool should be reviewed by the student interested in this technique (24).
3. Another procedure, mentioned by Van Riper after his discussion of other techniques, consists of the following: "If the consonants which require extra mouth pressure (*p-b; t-d; k-g; s-z; ch-j*) are those which are nasally distorted while the *r* and the *l* or *f* and *v* are quite adequate, we would feel that the closure was poor" (25). If the closure is poor, this could mean that the soft palate and pharyngeal wall are not meeting or closing off in the proper manner, and as a result speech may be distorted.
4. "Another technique which has been used to study nasality has consisted of obtaining oral and nasal sound pressure levels utilizing a microphone placed either in the nostril or in front of the nostril and in front of the mouth" (15).

Studies conducted in the senior author's laboratory have indicated that for subjects with complete velopharyngeal closure, the oral and nasal sound pressure levels would be essentially the same. When a velopharyngeal gap is present, the nasal SPL (sound pressure level) will be greater than the oral SPL (15).

Figure 3.1 shows an SPL tracing for a patient who has velopharyngeal closure. Figure 3.2 shows a tracing for a patient who does not have velopharyngeal closure. Note that more nasal sound pressure is present than oral sound pressure.

Radiography. One of the better methods for determining the presence or absence of velopharyngeal closure is cinefluorography (X-ray movies). The advantage of X-ray movies over the basic still X-ray film is that the movements of the palate and of the pharyngeal wall and other parts of the speech mechanism can be studied during speech production. Figure 3.3, a tracing made from a cinefluorography film, shows the palate meeting with the pharyngeal wall during speech production. Figure 3.4 shows another tracing when the palate lacks only 4mm of meeting with the back of the throat, and this may be considered a small velopharyngeal gap. In Figure 3.5 the tracing shows a velopharyngeal gap of 14mm. How these different types of velopharyngeal gaps relate to the habilitation procedures will be discussed later in this chapter.

The three methods just reviewed for studying the presence or absence of nasality and velopharyngeal competency may not be available for all speech pathologists who work with cleft-palate patients. The cinefluorography equipment and the oral and nasal sound-pressure equipment may be available only at a medical center. But the speech clinician can attempt the evaluation

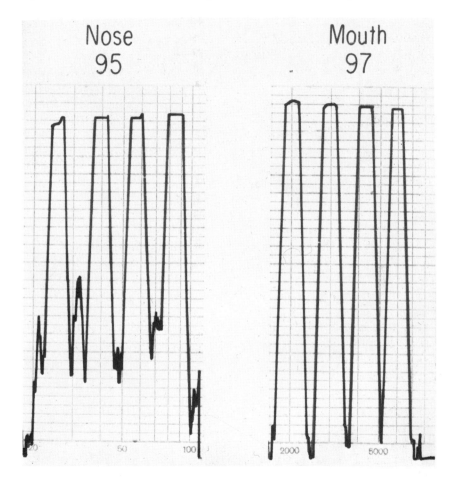

Fig. 3.1. Sound-pressure reading for patient with velopharyngeal closure

using the other methods described and, if necessary, he can ask for help from his colleagues at the medical center. As Westlake and Rutherford have so rightfully stated: "Consultation should not be a threat or source of embarrassment even to experienced and highly trained therapists. All should want another opinion on difficult cases" (19).

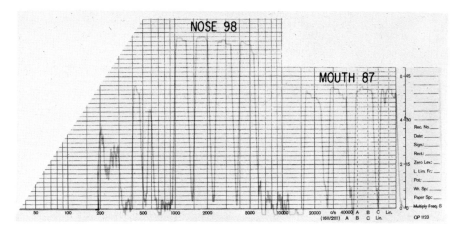

Fig. 3.2. Sound-pressure reading for patient without velopharyngeal closure

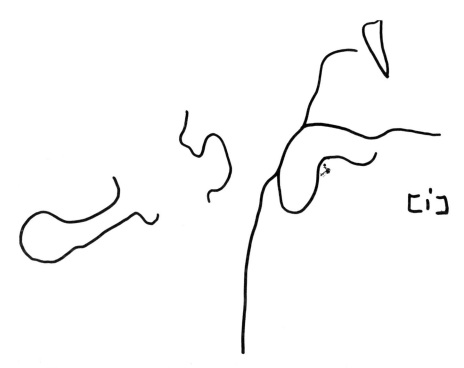

Fig. 3.3. Cinefluorography tracing showing complete velopharyngeal closure

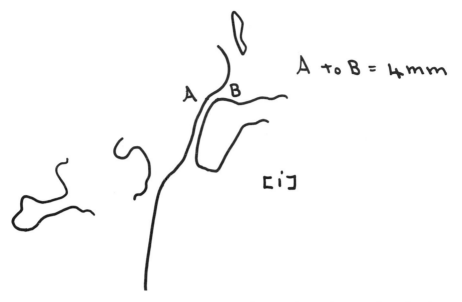

Fig. 3.4. Cinefluorography tracing showing a distance of 4mm between the soft palate and the pharyngeal wall

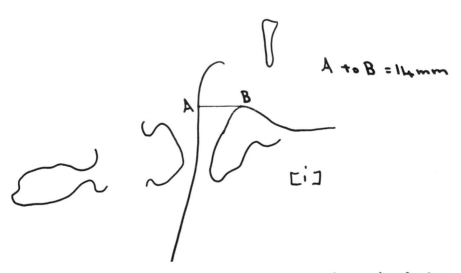

Fig. 3.5. Cinefluorography tracing showing a distance of 14mm between the soft palate and the pharyngeal wall

Therapy Procedures

Generally speaking, it can be assumed that the development of language is the primary concern with the cleft-palate child just as with any child. This means that the earliest or first activities are aimed at language development. Articulation is the next consideration. Accurate articulation enhances the intelligibility of speech and, thus, its usefulness for communication purposes. This hierarchy places therapy directed toward the elimination of nasality in third place. This means third place in the chronological order of emphasis, not in terms of importance. Actually, it is misleading to think in terms of such a division of therapy since all aspects of therapy can be taught somewhat simultaneously. Nasality is a major concern in therapy, but language must be developed before therapy can be engaged in to reduce nasality. Likewise, the elimination of nasality will not produce clear speech if poor articulation persists. Therapy for language stimulation and articulation will be dealt with later. The following are descriptions of techniques that can be employed to reduce nasality.

Visual Techniques. The clinician may want to try to teach the patient what takes place during velopharyngeal closure. Figures illustrating cinefluorography tracings of the palate and pharyngeal wall, such as those used in this book, can be employed. The clinician draws a picture of the soft palate and illustrates to the patient how it must move up and back to meet with the throat and help prevent sound from escaping into the nasal cavity. The clinician may borrow cinefluorography films from the medical center or university, showing them in slow motion, and again at regular speed, to help the patient and his parents understand how the soft palate should move.

The speech clinician also has the patient observe the palatal movement of another individual's palate during sustained phonation of /a/, *ah.* If cinefluorography films of the patient's palatal movement have been produced, these are shown to the patient as well as his parents.

Oral-mirrors, such as those used by dentists, are used to help the patient observe the palatal movements of the speech clinician working with him. Specially designed mirrors with attached lights are now available, and they can be used by the patient to observe his own palatal movements.

The therapy program will be enhanced if the patient has a thorough understanding of how his soft palate should function. The speech clinician should have the patient observe his palatal movements, utilizing the mirror with the light when certain sounds are produced. The patient also can observe certain raising and lowering aspects of his own palate and of his speech clinician's palate.

Auditory Techniques. Many hypernasal cleft-palate children realize that their speech is different from that of others but are not sure in what way.

The excess nasal resonance can be heard by the patient when a tape-recording of his speech is played. In helping him to understand, as well as in helping to correct this condition, ear-training is useful. "It is important, of course, to use the usual ear-training to identify the defectiveness of a given sound and to contrast it with the correct sound" (25). This does not indicate the standard ear-training for correct articulation. More will be discussed in this area later.

The speech clinician says a word, pauses a few seconds, and then has the patient repeat the word while it is being tape-recorded. Later he produces a short phrase, such as "Susie saw the silly sisters," pauses a few seconds, and then has the patient repeat the phrase. When the recording is played back, the patient listens to the difference between the sound of the clinician's voice and his own. After this procedure has been successfully utilized, the clinician has the patient try to imitate the clinician's voice or the voices of others who have normal voice quality. Standard recordings are utilized during this stage of therapy.

Another procedure is to have the patient listen to his own speech while his nostrils are open and then when they are closed, to help "establish auditory images of the sounds produced with and without nasal emission" (19).

With older cleft-palate children, ear-training can sometimes be worked on almost independently if the patient has access to a tape-recorder and is provided with proper instructions. The patient may be asked to make a five-minute talk on his favorite sport and have it recorded. When the recording is played back, the clinician and the patient judge which sounds or words were nasalized. They also may ask another individual, such as a teacher, school-counselor, or (at camp) a recreation specialist, to judge the tape to help determine which sounds or words are nasal. After the three judges have formulated a list of sounds or words that were perceived as being nasal, the patient practices producing these so as to eliminate as much hypernasality as possible. After careful practice another recording is produced and another judging procedure is conducted. Variations on this technique may be employed with the general objective of helping the patient to recognize when nasality is present and how, through ear-training, it can be alleviated.

Oral Air-Pressure Techniques. If a manometer is available, the patient can determine, with the help of his clinician, his oral air-pressure reading, with and without the nostrils manually occluded. If velopharyngeal closure is present, the reading with the nostrils occluded should be approximately the same as the reading when the nostrils are not occluded. The patient should practice trying to achieve the same readings with the nostrils not occluded as when the nostrils are occluded. After the advanced patient has learned how to use a manometer as a therapeutic device, he can work independently on exercises dealing with oral air pressure.

Another technique is to use an air paddle like the one employed by Bzoch (20). An air paddle can be made by cutting a 3 x 5 index card in the shape of a paddle. The paddle is held with two fingers and placed below the patient's nostrils. The patient is asked to produce sounds like /p, p, p/ or /b, b, b/, and the clinician and the patient watch the paddle to see if it moves. The paddle is then placed in front of the lips and the same procedure is repeated. The patient tries to produce these sounds without the paddle moving when it is under his nostrils, but he tries to move the paddle a great deal when it is in front of the lips. The advanced student can work on this technique by himself after he has learned it and its importance from his clinician.

Sucking Exercises.

In the past one technique we have used to aid in helping to promote a better velopharyngeal relationship has been sucking exercises. These exercises are initiated a year or so after palatal surgery and consist of the child trying to hold a small piece of paper on the bottom of a straw by the suction. The child attempts to hold the small piece of paper to the bottom of the straw for longer periods of time as the exercises continue (21).

The study (26) dealing with various aspects of this technique should be reviewed. With exercises, one of the main requirements is good motivation. If the child is not properly motivated to carry out his exercises and does them only sporadically, the overall results achieved will probably be limited.

Dental Prosthesis

Two types of prosthetic aids are usually utilized: (1) a palatal lift or stimulator and (2) a dental obturator.

Palatal Lift or Stimulator.

This palatal lift or stimulator may prove helpful to the patient whose velopharyngeal gap is not too large. It is described as a prosthetic device

made of acrylic which covers the hard palate and has an extension which fits against the velum. The palatal stimulator, similar to a palatal lift, differs as a prosthetic device from the speech bulb or obturator in that the stimulator extends only to the velum and fits against it in a rest position to stimulate movement away from the device. The obturator extends into the pharyngeal area to provide an adjunct to velopharyngeal valving (27).

When the cleft-palate team is thinking in terms of a palatal stimulator, a number of factors must be considered.

A patient whose velum appears to have adequate length but lacks necessary mobility for elevation to establish contact with the pharyngeal wall, and who exhibits a small to medium velopharyngeal (V-P) gap will probably be the most appropriate candidate for a stimulator. However, this technique of therapy has been used in cases with whom there are concomitant complications making other forms of therapy impractical (27).

Basically, when the soft palate shows fairly good mobility and the velopharyngeal gap is not too large, the palatal stimulator should be attempted. When the velopharyngeal distance is large and a prosthesis is to be employed, the dental obturator should be attempted. Figure 3.6 shows a palatal stimulator in use.

Dental Obturator. The dental obturator, like the palatal lift or stimulator, may be made of plastic and fits around the molars. As Yules points out,

> both the dental obturator and the palatal lift depend on teeth for support. Given adequate teeth, healthy gingivae, adequate occlusion, and good hygiene and motivation, prostheses can prove helpful in the secondary correction of velopharyngeal incompetence—especially in older patients with large gaps and/or in postcancer surgical patients (44).

While the palatal lift or stimulator fits against the soft palate, the obturator fits behind the soft palate and helps fill in the space or gap between the soft palate and the pharyngeal wall. At the senior author's clinic, the obturator

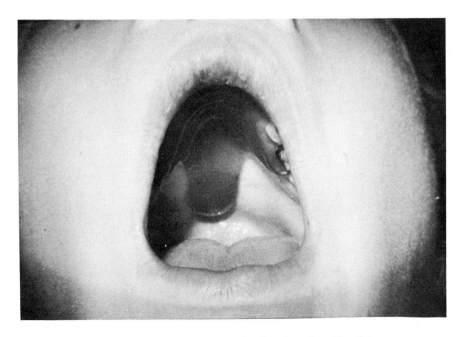

Fig. 3.6. A palatal stimulator fitted against the soft palate

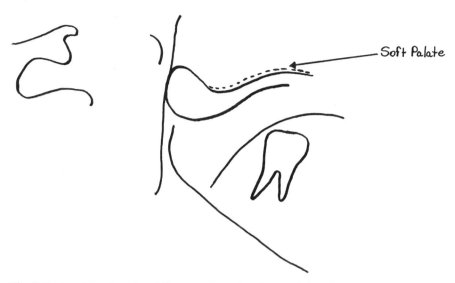

Fig. 3.7. An obturator placed between the soft palate and the pharyngeal wall to help prevent speech from escaping into the nose

has been used successfully with adults with unrepaired clefts of the palate and also with postcancer-surgery patients. In addition, the obturator has been used with patients who had either a paralyzed soft palate or pharyngeal wall. Figure 3.7 is a sketch showing an obturator, which fits between the soft palate and the pharyngeal wall, as opposed to the stimulator, which fits against the soft palate, as shown in Figure 3.6. Roberts (28) and Beder (29) provide information on obturators and prostheses that may be of interest to the student concerned with this aspect of cleft-palate habilitation.

Secondary Surgery

In some patients, even after primary palatal surgery, the palate may not be long enough to meet with the pharyngeal wall (throat) during speech. If surgery is considered to be the best means of coping with this problem, then two of the most popular methods are (1) palatal pushback procedures, whereby the soft palate is lengthened surgically and (2) the pharyngeal flap, whereby tissue is taken from the pharyngeal wall and attached to the soft palate. The tissue may be taken high (superiorly based flap), as shown in Part *A* of Figure 3.8, or low in the pharyngeal area, as shown in Part *B* of the same figure. It is beyond the scope of this book to go into the details of these surgical procedures, but the following references should be studied by students interested in this aspect of surgery: Massengill (15), Yules (30), and Converse (31). Secondary palatal surgery should be considered only after

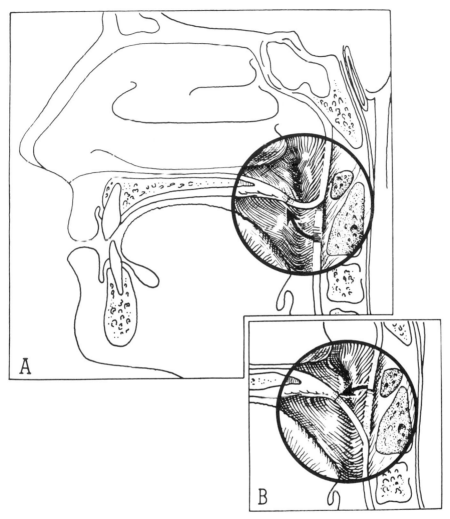

Fig. 3.8. *A*, a superiorly based pharyngeal flap; *B*, an inferiorly based pharyngeal flap

detailed studies are carried out by the appropriate members of the cleft-palate team.

Articulation

Probably the most unique speech problem experienced by the cleft-palate child is nasality, but certainly the problems of articulation are significantly associated with this condition. Speech sounds may be substituted, distorted, or omitted, and some unneeded extra sounds may be added. The anatomical

condition of the soft palate, hard palate, alveolar ridge, and lips, and irregu-
larities in the position of the teeth (as well as absent or extra teeth), can all
influence the child's articulation (21).

McWilliams (32), in her study dealing with intelligibility of cleft-palate
speech, pointed out that her findings support the views of Harkins and Baker
(33) that correcting poor articulation would be more beneficial in speech
therapy than any other procedure available. She also pointed out "that a
positive relationship exists between consonant articulation errors and ratings
of nasality as well as between intelligibility and ratings of nasality" (32). It is
hoped that the cleft-palate child will be seen by the cleft-palate team at regular
intervals and that the speech pathologist will counsel with the parents regarding speech and language stimulation, as mentioned elsewhere in this book.
Some children with repaired clefts do not have an articulation problem, but
many do, even though a proper home speech and language program has been
provided. Articulation problems range from very mild to very severe. Two
speech articulation problems often encountered by the cleft-palate patient are
the glottal stop and the pharyngeal fricative.

Glottal Stop

The glottal stop has been defined as a "tiny cough-like sound produced by
the sudden release of a pulse of voiced or unvoiced air from the vocal folds"
(25) and is transcribed phonetically /ʔ/. The vocal folds "have been drawn
together by hypertension in the laryngeal muscles" (16). Morley indicated that
the glottal stop

> is often used by a cleft palate patient as a substitute for plosive sounds which,
> due to the defect, cannot be made correctly, the patient feeling subconsciously
> that this is the only position where the breath stream can be interrupted to
> obtain the requisite pressure for a plosive sound (16).

The glottal stop can be substituted for consonant sounds and is "usually
substituted for any or all of the plosive consonants /p/, /b/, /t/, /d/, /k/ and
/g/" (16). In the experience of both authors, the glottal stop, in patients who
have had their palates repaired late in life, is one of the speech problems
hardest to alleviate. The glottal stop provides an acoustic cue that definitely
distinguishes an individual's speech as being different. Many adult cleft-palate
patients describe the glottal stop as the speech impairment they most want to
eliminate.

Pharyngeal Fricatives

Often, when there are glottal stops, there will also be pharyngeal fricatives.
Here the production of plosive consonants is usually accompanied by the
"substitution of some fricative sounds made in the pharynx or larynx for the

normal fricatives /s/, /z/, /sh ($\int$)/, /th (θ, $\eth$)/, /zh (z)/, /f/, and /v/" (16). The /s/ sound is the one most frequently produced in this manner (16).

It is impossible to outline an articulation-therapy program appropriate for every cleft-palate patient, but the following techniques and procedures should be considered when appropriate.

Adequate Jaw, Lip, and Tongue Positions during Speech Production. The authors have seen cleft-palate children who speak with their mouths barely open, and as a partial result much of their speech comes out of their noses. The cleft-palate patient should be taught to open his mouth wide when he talks (though not abnormally wide), so as to direct more speech out of the mouth and less out of the nose. The clinician may have to use exaggerated wide-mouth openings at the beginning of therapy to emphasize this factor and later the normal mouth opening after the child understands what is expected. At the Duke University summer speech camp, this point is illustrated by means of a picture of a clown with a mouth that is adjustable to different degrees of opening. Mirror drills are also used for this technique.

The cleft-palate patient may have a tendency to show very little lip mobility. Lip exercises to provide for greater lip motion may prove helpful. The lips are very important in promoting a wider mouth opening. Without adequate lip mobility, many of the labial sounds, such as /b/, /p/, /v/, and /f/, may be distorted. Since the phonetic placement is easy to see, the clinician can illustrate how lips move to produce labial sounds by using a mirror or having the patient observe him.

In Berry and Eisenson's discussion of speech habilation in cleft palate, it is pointed out that "in the majority of these children we find that the tongue habitually is retracted in the mouth, producing a high-riding dorsum, and that the blade and tip are inflexible" (34). The child may develop the habit of carrying the dorsum or back of the tongue high before the palate is surgically closed. This habit may develop as a technique the child learns from helping to close off the open cleft. The child may continue this habit even after the palate is closed. Some cinefluorography films have shown the tongue coming back and pushing the soft palate so as to raise and move the soft palate back toward the pharyngeal wall.

The tongue position during speech production should be studied carefully, and the clinician should explain to the patient the correct tongue placement for the different sounds. The importance of correct phonetic placement cannot be overemphasized. Exercises for the tongue tip and tongue blade should be carried out. Poor tongue positions can produce defective speech for the cleft-palate patient even if his palate is functioning properly. Van Riper has written that "exercises for increasing the mobility of the tongue include sensitization of the tonguetip, curling, grooving, lifting, lowering, thrusting, arching, tapping, sustaining postures, pressing, scraping, fluttering, and many others" (25).

Directing the Breath Stream Out of the Mouth instead of the Nose.   Sucking exercises have already been listed as a technique that can aid in promoting a better velopharyngeal relationship. Some have indicated lung exercises for this purpose. Blowing exercises can be used to some degree to help the patient become aware of directing the air stream out of the mouth. Blowing small amounts of confetti or a ping-pong ball can be utilized for this purpose; so can a manometer drill.

Breath Control.   As in any speech situation, proper breath control is important. "Many cleft-palate cases require training in breath control for speech. Their breathing records show many instances of air wastage, speaking on residual air, opposition, and staircase breathing" (25).

Using the Various Techniques during Conversational Speech.   The procedures already discussed, such as directing the breath stream through the mouth, adequate phonetic placement, large mouth opening, and so on, must not only be carried out during individual drills but must become a part of the patient's speech pattern during conversational speech. The authors have observed patients who could name each of these techniques and demonstrate them, but forgot to utilize the techniques when they started conversational speech dealing with other matters. This is why it is important to try to make those techniques that work well for the patient matters of habit. At the Duke University summer speech camp, one technique emphasized with the repaired-cleft-palate patient is therapy sessions based on free-flowing conversational speech. These therapy sessions are a part of the total therapeutic program. In connected speech the child tells about his favorite sport, his vacation last summer, or the talent show or skit night that may be taking place during his stay at the camp. If the child can carry over into conversational speech the techniques that have been taught him during the formal therapy sessions, progress has been achieved. See the Appendix for further suggestions of specific therapeutic techniques that can be employed.

Chapter 4

The Role of the Speech Pathologist

The work of the speech pathologist can be divided into two areas: counseling and therapy. There are times when the activity is clearly defined and falls neatly into one or the other category; other times it is difficult to determine where the counseling ends and the therapy begins. Much of the counseling is directed to the parents, but it also involves the patient—especially the older patient. Although the speech pathologist is not a psychologist and recognizes his limitations as a counselor, clearly he must be aware of the areas in which counseling will be a necessary part of his service.

Counseling

Working under ideal circumstances—that is, with a cleft-palate team—the role of the speech pathologist would begin with the birth of the cleft lip/palate baby. This is not always the case. Sometimes the child is not seen by a speech specialist until he reaches school age. In any event, the initial conference should be devoted to orienting the parents to their long-term responsibilities and to answering their questions, whether verbalized or not, concerning their cleft-palate child.

Regardless of when the first meeting between parents and speech pathologist takes place, it should be an educational one. Although it can be assumed that the parents have already been given an explanation of their child's deformity, and of its cause and treatment, it is safe to assume that a further explanation by the speech pathologist will not be overly redundant. Parents suffering from the initial shock of discovering the cleft condition in their newborn might have been unable to comprehend all that was told them; some of the initial explanation might have been purposely "glossed over"; some of it might have been vague or inaccurate; much of what was initially explained may have been forgotten by the parents; and sometimes repetition is desirable for better understanding. Unless the speech pathologist actively engages in the educational aspect of the cleft condition, many parental questions may go unanswered. It is best to take nothing for granted and to start at the beginning, but in the explanation carefully consider the educational level of the parents.

45

With all parents it should be the goal of the speech specialist to keep the explanation simple. He should not try to impress them with technical terms or complicated recitations. Perhaps the greatest mark of true genius is the ability to explain a complicated subject in simple terms. If the parent does not understand the explanation, then little has been gained by the exercise; indeed, time and perhaps rapport may have been lost.

The speech pathologist should remember that, although a cleft lip and palate are particularly disfiguring for the baby and alarming for the mother to see for the first time, there is usually a rapid dissipation of the initial shock felt by the parents. Unlike the parents of mentally retarded or cerebral-palsy children, these parents have a child whose disorder is remediable, and information about remediation was given to them when they were first told about the condition. The fact that remedial procedures exist may help to allay some of their anxiety (35).

To participate adequately as a member of the cleft-palate team, the speech pathologist needs basic information relative to the patient's condition and to the parents' attitudes, as well as training in dealing with such situations and empathy for the people involved. Since the clefting condition is an anomaly of the oral mechanism and involves both preventive and habilitative procedures in speech and language development, the speech pathologist assumes a major role in the total habilitation program. Kallaus (36) has suggested five goals for the speech pathologist in counseling with parents of cleft-palate children:

1. Establishing a link with the parents to facilitate communication with them.
2. Giving accurate, consistent, and objective information concerning the anomaly's cause and character.
3. Revising parental attitudes toward the deformity.
4. Reducing anxieties concerning the child's future.
5. Increasing parental understanding of, as well as cooperation in, the total clinic process—especially the speech and language.

Establish Rapport

For any type of counseling to be successful, the counselor must first establish rapport—make the parents feel that they can confide in him. Once the initial shock at having a cleft lip/palate child has been expressed, many mothers begin to feel that negative feelings are bad and must be disclaimed. Unexpressed feelings of inadequacy or guilt for having produced a congenitally defective baby, or feelings of rejection toward an unacceptable offspring, may be internalized. The feelings may be present, but the mother verbalizes different attitudes. An empathetic speech pathologist is able to create an accepting atmosphere in which the parent will feel able to express feelings and ask previously hidden questions.

Provide Information

Although other members of the cleft-palate team may have already discussed the cause and character of the child's condition with the parents, the speech pathologist should also make this explanation. This repetition will help to reconstruct many facts that may have been forgotten and to clarify points that may have been misunderstood or omitted. Explanations must be presented in understandable terms, and it must be remembered that visual aids are important tools. Drawings, mirror self-examinations, textbooks, films, slides, and verbal explanations with simplified terminology can all be used to explain:

1. The arching of the palatal shelves.
2. The positioning of the premaxilla and action of the velum.
3. The double-sling functioning of the muscles necessary for quick lift of the soft palate.
4. The strong contact of the velum with the pharyngeal wall necessary to prevent nasal escape of sound (37).

With reference to the cause, it is well to point out to the parents that exact causes are not yet known and may never be known for their particular child. In removing feelings of guilt concerning the cause, it is important to emphasize the chance factor. Even with these explanations, however, parents may harbor previous beliefs concerning the cause. It is important for the speech pathologist to probe the parents' feelings and beliefs about the cause of their child's cleft. Because a genetic explanation may not have been sufficient, parents may have resorted to fantasies (38) reflecting serious guilt feelings or superstitions, cultural attitudes, or folklore beliefs (39). Although parents, even well-educated ones, may accept the medical explanation for cleft-palate causation at one level, they frequently cannot forget and cannot disregard the relevancy of many of the "old wives tales" that they have heard.

Although providing accurate information is a goal of the speech specialist, it is not always possible to discount these earlier beliefs. It may be meaningless to some parents to tell them that their superstitions and folk beliefs are illogical, irrational, and unscientific; therefore, it may be necessary to allow such beliefs to exist. After providing the scientific information, the therapist should accept the parents with sympathetic understanding and get on with the business of providing the best habilitation program possible for the child. It should be recognized that guilt is not always neurotic or harmful, and that it can be used as a positive motivating force in the treatment process (39).

Revise Attitudes

The revision of parental attitudes toward the deformity is a worthwhile goal since it is assumed that parental attitudes are conveyed to the child and affect his development. One of the parents' major areas of concern is the child's appearance. The speech pathologist can remind the parents that surgical procedures will increasingly improve the cosmetic appearance of the cleft and the functional ability of the palate in speech.

Parents must take an objective and realistic attitude toward the child and his handicap, for it will be their responsibility to help in his future adjustment. The cleft-palate child does not inherently know that he is different from others. He acquires this awareness from the feedback provided by others within his environment—parents, family, neighbors, professionals, and strangers. The type of preparation he is given for these responses will affect his psychological reactions to them and to his defect. If parents fail to accept the child's deformity openly and unemotionally, and fail to prepare him to do the same, the first feedback about his defect that he receives from others may lead to feelings of self-pity or disgust. In such a situation, the child may feel that the anomaly is characteristic of his entire self (35).

The revision of parental attitudes, then, is not an end in itself. The goal is to prepare the child to face his "difference" without losing his feelings of self-worth.

Reduce Anxieties

The reduction of parental anxieties has a direct influence on fostering a good mother-child relationship. Anxieties can result in fear of handling the child, failure to engage in the normal cuddling and cooing that mothers commonly do with a newborn, and perhaps strained relations with other members of the family. Instruction in how to feed the child, in how to stimulate him vocally, in the importance of cuddling and playing with him, are all aspects of developing a good mother-child relationship.

Parental anxieties also involve concerns for the child's future. The subject of mental retardation may arise, for there is often a feeling that "the child whose head is damaged from the outside may be damaged from the inside too" (38). A simple recitation of the statistical incidence of mental retardation among the cleft-palate population should not be considered any more sufficient than simply referring the parents to a psychologist. The speech pathologist should discover what the parent means by "mental retardation" and then be prepared to discuss the subject with reference to the specific child. Referring the child for psychological testing may be a part of the overall therapy procedure, but at this particular point in the parent-counseling activities, the actual assessment of the child's I.Q. score is not the goal.

Parents often express anxieties relative to the child's ability to learn speech. Parents should understand that the development of expressive speech may be delayed, that intelligible speech may not be developed until all the surgery has been performed, and that speech therapy may be needed for a relatively long period of time; they must also understand that the child's ability to understand verbal communication is in no way delayed and, therefore, requires much stimulation. Emphasis on the many sources of language stimulation should be given, and parents should be helped to understand the child's need for this stimulation in order to learn in areas such as gaining information, socialization with others, and the development of intellect.

Counseling should include reassurance that adequate surgical correction, proper environmental motivation and stimulation, and good speech training all combine to promise a good prognosis for normal speech. Along with this should be some information suggesting that the typical adult with a cleft palate is usually married, gainfully employed, and in general a useful, contributing member of society (35). It may be in order to suggest that the parent is unaware of the existence of successfully rehabilitated cleft-palate individuals because their corrected conditions are not apparent. Only the unsuccessful ones—those, perhaps, who did not receive adequate early attention—are readily identifiable.

Understand Total Clinic Process

Parental participation and cooperation in a program of remediation are essential if optimum results are to be obtained; however, this participation must be directed. The main areas of concern to the speech pathologist are speech and language development as "parents are going to teach speech (and language), either consciously or unconsciously, and their teaching is likely to be harmful if not directed" (37). As already suggested, parents need a simple but thorough explanation of how language and articulation are acquired. Simple suggestions relative to socializing with the infant, holding him so that he can see the parent's face, directing his attention to the parent's facial movements and sound-making, will all lead to needed imitative behavior in the child.

Parents must not be misled into believing that the child will have perfect speech as soon as his palate is surgically closed. Bad habits may persist; velopharyngeal closure may be impossible; and dental malocclusions may distort productions. To prevent parents from labeling the child as "lazy," the speech pathologist should explain the conditions that are prerequisite to good speech. Parents need information about what they should expect from the child. For instance, with a child who is unable to effect velopharyngeal closure, the admonition to "try harder" to eliminate nasal emission may result in the child's trying harder all right, but the result will be undesirable.

He may exhibit even more nasal emission by exerting more effort, or he may learn to employ the glottal stop to substitute for difficult consonants. In short, adequate surgical management, together with a dedicated and united effort of speech pathologist, parents, and child, will produce the best possible results.

Therapy

There is usually little or no need for a speech pathologist to work directly with a child whose cleft involves only the lip. If the child with a repaired cleft lip exhibits an upper lip that is immobile, tight, and short, he may have problems with the "production of labio-dental sounds such as /f/ and /v/," and possibly other sounds (16). If such is the case, this information should be presented to the referring cleft-palate team for its consideration and recommendations. Basically, if the patient has only a cleft lip and the surgery for this condition is successful, there will not usually be any speech problem. Therapy discussions, therefore, will involve individuals with a cleft palate either with or without an associated cleft of the lip. When the term *cleft palate* is used in the following discussion, this will be the intended meaning.

Morley (16) suggests that therapy can be broadly divided into three stages:

1. Therapy for children under four years of age.
2. Therapy for children over four years of age.
3. Therapy for older children and adults.

Therapy for Children Under Four Years of Age

Therapy for the cleft-palate child in the infant age-group is basically performed by the parents (usually the mother or mother surrogate). This indicates that the speech pathologist's services are directed toward the parents. "Verbal communication commensurate with the child's ability can be encouraged by introduction, during infancy, of activities to promote the development of language and speech skills" (37). Such a program, although preceded by parent counseling relative to normal speech-motivating activities, should begin around eighteen to twenty-four months of age, or shortly after the child begins to talk. See the discussion of therapy for children over four years of age, below, for suggestions on motivating speech.

It is appropriate to keep certain principles of therapy in mind when working with the very young child or when giving the parents direction in their speech-stimulation program.

Principles of Learning Are Not Unlike Those of the Normal Child

Speech is learned, and most children are taught by their parents. Since this is done primarily on a rather hit-or-miss basis, and since most children learn to talk adequately, it must be realized that most parents tend to do a fairly good job. It can also be said that most children tend to sort of "catch it on the wing." For a child with a handicap, that makes the learning of speech a bit difficult, and parents may need some help in organizing their teaching of speech. This does not mean that their child learns by a different set of principles; rather, his instruction must be clearer and sharper.

Therapy Should Be Provided in an Accepting Atmosphere

The therapist should provide an accepting atmosphere in order to demonstrate for the parent the setting in which speech stimulation should take place. This is essential for the child. It is also helpful for mothers who are tense or overconcerned about their role as therapist, mothers who are overindulgent or overprotective, and mothers who feel that learning only takes place in a rigid or highly structured classroom-type setting.

Therapy Is Most Effective in a One-to-One Relationship

Small children do not play together. They may play in the proximity of another child, but they play alone. It follows that therapy for the very young child is most profitable when given individually.

Parents Should Participate in Therapy

For the very young child it is usually recommended that the parent participate in the therapy situation. There are several reasons for this. First, the young child is usually more reluctant to be separated from his mother; thus, parent participation adds a security to the therapy situation that the child may need in order to profit optimally from it. Second, if the mother is essentially to be the therapist carrying out the demonstrated therapy activities, then it is helpful for her to participate in the activities. This enables the parent to become familiar with the tools and procedures employed. Likewise, it gives the therapist an opportunity to observe the mother working with the child, her ability to carry out the activities, and her understanding of the directions that she has been given.

Therapy Sessions Must Be Geared to Play Activities

The very young child profits little from short formal sessions unless these are strictly demonstration sessions in which the mother is given an outline to follow and shown the procedures involved in the many activities included in her outline. The young child has a short attention span and activities must be changed frequently; yet he is capable of long play periods. The long session allows freedom for the child to engage in spontaneous vocalizations and for the therapist to capitalize on the child's use of speech; the short formal session cannot be structured so freely.

Activities Must Be Simple, Repetitious, and Socializing

Young children respond to rhyming, rhythmic activities, familiar stories, and physical contact. Nursery rhymes, clapping games, and social activities ranging from "peek-a-boo" to "tea party," provide verbal stimulation.

Activities Should Be Developmental in Organization

The entire therapy program must be planned so that the activities follow a developmental rather than an incidental sequence. There are many procedures that may be engaged in, but if they are a part of the therapy program they must have a purpose grounded in the developmental sequence of language learning.

Therapy for Children over Four Years of Age

If early directed therapy provided by the mother has been successful, and if surgical management has been effective, then perhaps no further therapy will be needed. If, however, there is still a speech or voice problem (which seems to be the rule rather than the exception), the speech pathologist will have the child in regular speech therapy. A child of this age is usually able to cooperate and profit from an organized and more structured therapy program. The mother's presence may still be desirable, either as a participant or as an observer, since her help with daily practice at home will still be indicated. With effective handling at this time, normal to near normal speech is often achieved before the child enters school.

As nearly normal speech as possible before the child enters school is a desirable goal, since both social and educational consequences are to be considered. For most children, additional progress can be expected when they enter school. The added stimulus from peers, together with the visual cues and the emphasis placed on sounds in most instructional reading-readiness programs, provides impetus for further improvement in speech and language.

Therapy for Older Children and Adults

With older children, therapy will doubtless be more structured. The therapist may have to rely strictly on his relationship with the client since parents may not accompany these children, and it may be necessary to provide short daily therapy sessions. For the adult, however, therapy sessions may be less frequent since a properly motivated adult will usually maintain carry-over from one therapy session to another for a longer time span and will be diligent in home assignments. Adult patients must be properly motivated; therapy will face a poor prognosis unless the speech pathologist is able to motivate the patient.

Group Versus Individual Therapy

Although it is assumed that therapy with the young child is best administered individually, the same may not be true for the child past four or five years of age. Group therapy has certain advantages, which can perhaps be described as (1) economy in time and (2) improved outlook for the child.

Unless time is profitably spent, the first-listed advantage could be a false one. Sometimes so-called group therapy is simply individual therapy presented serially. Good group therapy, on the other hand, involves the entire group and is truly economical with time since a greater number of patients can be treated at the same time. This factor is further enhanced by the tendency of children to learn from their peers so that therapy seems to move faster with more progress. The advantage, then, would be one of more children making better progress.

Group therapy provides an opportunity for the cleft-palate child to find himself in the company of others with similar problems, some of whom may have problems more severe than his. From these contacts the child discovers that he is not the only person with a cleft palate. This helps him to understand many things, including the possibility that his speech is unintelligible. He is also provided with an opportunity to observe other children making progress and to realize that progress is rewarding.

There is evidence that it may be necessary to supplement group therapy with individual therapy, and this appears to be the most ideal arrangement. For children living in thinly populated areas, however, group therapy may not be possible. Medical specialities and the needed dental services may also be unavailable locally. One method of providing a concerted therapeutic program is to bring a number of cleft-palate children together during summer vacation at a summer speech camp like the ones at Duke University and Florida State University. Anyone interested in such a summer program should contact his state's crippled-children's department or rehabilitation center, requesting information about the availability of such a camp for his child. These camps provide an opportunity for controlled environment and intensive speech therapy for the child, along with medical and dental attention (37).

Chapter 5

Problems Associated with Cleft Palate

Although the cleft condition is a problem in itself, this is not the only problem of the cleft-palate child. His associated problems include those of feeding, respiration, intelligence, psychological adjustment, social competence, dentition, hearing, and speech. Perhaps some of these areas need a more thorough investigation by the speech pathologist than others, but all should be considered as potentially significant.

Feeding

Feeding has already been mentioned and a reference was cited for instruction in feeding procedures (13). Suffice it to say here that the obvious difficulty in maintaining the pressure needed for sucking is of immediate concern to parent and physician. The cleft lip/palate baby is as hungry as any other youngster, but he lacks the mechanism for normal sucking. Special feeders are usually employed with the infant until surgical repair of the lip has been effected. The lip is generally closed quite soon following birth, depending on the health of the infant. For a healthy baby this may be accomplished before he and his mother leave the hospital. If the baby has some other complication, closure may be delayed. The palate will be closed considerably later, and the problem of an open palate complicates feeding since it allows the milk to flow into the nasal cavity. Again, a special feeding apparatus may be needed to counteract this difficulty.

Respiration

Special breathing problems may be encountered. The deficiency or collapse of the nasal crura or deviation of the septum may cause mouth breathing. The deficiency or malformation of the bony structures of the nose may obstruct the nasal passage, resulting in mouth breathing. Children tend to have more upper respiratory infections than adults, and cleft-palate children have more than the average noncleft child. Breathing may be noisy, shallow, and irregular because of nasal obstructions.

Intelligence

Although many early studies indicated a positive relationship between cleft palate and intellectual impairment, more recent studies do not necessarily support this observation. It is true that scores on traditional I.Q. tests are somewhat lower for the cleft-palate population than for the population as a whole. Closer investigation reveals that verbal scores are lower than performance scores. This should be judged in light of the indication that language development is somewhat delayed in the cleft-palate child; thus his use of language may result in a slight downward skewing of I.Q. scores. Too, studies of mentally retarded populations indicate a higher incidence of cleft-palate individuals in the mentally retarded population than in the population as a whole. This too would skew the scores toward the lower limits. Yet, with these two considerations in mind, it is noted that the lower intelligence scores are not present at a statistically significant level.

There are two important considerations here: (1) It should not be assumed that because a child has a cleft palate there is a likelihood of his being mentally retarded. (2) If he is mentally retarded, the speech pathologist should be aware of this fact in order to make a more accurate assessment of the prognosis for the child's speech correction and to plan appropriate therapy procedures.

Some behaviors tend to lead to a misdiagnosis of mental retardation. For example, if a child's speech and language development are delayed, this may contribute to the erroneous conclusion that he is mentally retarded. Also, handicapped children are often treated differently from nonhandicapped children, and this may result in social immaturity. Again, this may cause the child to appear less intelligent than he actually is. Overprotection may result in a child's having limited experiences, which in turn gives the same impression. These are only examples, but they serve to point up the possibility of misdiagnosis. It is important for the speech pathologist to know if the child is truly mentally retarded; but judgment must be made carefully. Hunches or guesses are no substitute for objective data. Finally, remember that the speech pathologist's consideration of mental retardation as a significant concern is not unique for the cleft-palate patient.

Psychological Adjustment

It has frequently been asserted that the cleft-palate person tends to exhibit certain personality traits; but "research dealing with the psychological and social aspects of cleft palate has not convincingly demonstrated that children with cleft palate are psychologically different from unaffected children" (37). However, certain problems are encountered, and the speech pathologist should be aware of them.

First, any handicapped child tends to split his family into two groups—the mother and the handicapped child constituting one group, and the father and the rest of the children making up the second group (37). One must not overlook the feelings of the parents, who have looked forward to the birth of a perfect baby. Feelings of hurt, disappointment, resentment, guilt, and shame must be considered sympathetically. Along with these personal feelings of ill fate, parents also experience concern and often bewilderment over such fundamental questions as "How will he eat?" and "Will he be able to talk?" Other concerns involve the child's appearance, whether or not surgery is indicated on such a young child, the expense involved, the reaction of siblings, and the chance of subsequent children being similarly deformed. Some questions, which may not be voiced but nonetheless constitute real concerns, relate to the child's intellectual potential, the reaction of family and friends, and most especially the effect that the birth of this child will have on the parents' relationships with each other.

These are not indications that parents of cleft-palate children have personalities different from parents of normal children; rather, these are normal reactions that have no impetus without an event like the birth of a child with a deformity. The feelings are real and the parents may need counseling; but they may not seek counseling directly. Sometimes the speech pathologist is the first person to become aware of some of these feelings. If so, he should be prepared.

A consideration of psychological problems must not be confined solely to the parents. Those of the child must not be overlooked. Although research indicates that cleft-palate youngsters are essentially normal children in their emotional development, it must be remembered that they have encountered some influences that the normal child does not encounter. For this reason, the cleft-palate child may well have some psychological reactions to his handicap and these merit consideration. First of all, he may become sensitive about his appearance and speech. Obviously, if his surgery has resulted in a normal-appearing face and in normal-sounding speech, this will not happen. If, however, surgery was delayed, or if it was insufficiently rehabilitative to effect normalcy, the child will experience some emotional reactions to his handicap as he reaches preadolescence. It is, therefore, a goal of corrective surgery and speech therapy to prevent this from becoming a major handicap.

The psychologist may be helpful in aiding the parents and the child to guard against feelings of rejection and guilt, but in some cases the speech pathologist and the social worker do much along these lines. The child needs help, also, in learning to adjust to his appearance. Here again the psychologist may be aided by other members of the team in accomplishing this, as well as in helping the child to develop emotional toughness and in motivating him to develop maximally efficient speech.

With reference to the child's social development, it is difficult to generalize because of the many variables that may help or hinder this adjustment. It can probably be assumed, however, that if the child developed speech at a slower rate than the normal child, he may likewise have a somewhat retarded rate of social development. This should not be interpreted as an inevitable outcome, nor should it be interpreted as a permanent social retardation. Usually, although somewhat slower in social development, cleft-palate children, all other factors being equal, catch up or reach the average level of social maturity of other children.

Dentition

The very nature of the structural abnormality of a cleft palate suggests the accompanying problem of abnormal dentition. With misplaced or missing tooth buds, the child may have too few teeth, jumbled teeth, poorly developed teeth, and malocclusion. In addition to the structural problem, there is frequently the additional problem of dental health. There is a high degree of tooth decay among the cleft-palate population. Some of this problem arises from the malocclusion; some of it arises from the feeding problem, which encourages a prolonged soft diet. Frequently such diets are high in glucose and low in protein, thus leading to more tooth decay.

Adding to the significance of maintaining dental health and the problem of doing so is the necessity for dental braces and prosthetic devices. Teeth must be maintained in order to have attachments for such appliances, but these appliances contribute to the problem of keeping teeth clean and healthy. Furthermore, orthodontic braces cause difficulty in eating certain foods and may therefore add to the poor eating habits.

Responsibility for the dental program must be accepted by both the child and his parents. Support by the speech pathologist will enhance their acceptance of this responsibility.

Hearing

Cleft-palate children tend to have a bilateral conductive type of hearing loss. An investigation of the implications of this suggests that these children need close monitoring of their hearing acuity and hearing health. At birth, over 90 percent of cleft-palate infants have a watery fluid in the middle ear (40). Initially this fluid is not infected, and there are no signs of pain, fever, or hearing loss (41), but if this fluid is allowed to remain untreated, subsequent complications may arise. The earlier condition, known as serous otitis media, then becomes chronic otitis media, and there may be resultant perforation of the tympanic membrane (ear drum), pain, and a hearing loss. Further deterioration of the condition, known as the adhesive stage, will result in still more hearing loss and, if unchecked, can develop into infection of the mastoid bone, cholesteatoma, or death.

Evidence of the presence of the initial ear disease, however, is so subtle that parents may be unaware of the indications, which may include persistent ear rubbing, fluctuating fever, and a periodic hearing loss. The latter condition indicates that one hearing test or hearing screening may not be sufficient evidence on which to base a conclusion that a child has normal hearing. Very young cleft-palate children with serous otitis media may have a periodic loss no greater than thirty decibels, but since speech loudness level is approximately thirty to forty decibels (42), this is a significant loss in terms of speech and language learning. It may be significant, too, in terms of the kind of language hearing to which the child is exposed. Soft, endearing, "I love you" type of talk may go unheard; whereas louder admonishments of "No, no!" and "Stop that!" may be heard. It can be assumed that a child with such fluctuating loss misses some speech for at least periods of time.

If mild infections and resultant hearing losses are not controlled, they may become worse and even permanent. Yules found that over 50 percent of all cleft-palate patients had a permanent conductive hearing loss (40). Such a loss of thirty decibels or more affects the quality of speech. It has been found that 90 percent of cleft-palate patients with this type of loss were hypernasal (42), while only 55 percent with normal hearing were hypernasal. Those with a thirty-decibel to forty-decibel loss were hypernasal even after successful surgery, with no physical reason for nasality except that the hearing was not efficient enough for proper monitoring of speech. These cleft-palate patients cannot hear the subtle differences to correct their own speech; therefore, a speech pathologist must use other than auditory means to correct the nasality. Visual and sensory cues must supplement the usual auditory training. Although these are good techniques to use with a patient who has a permanent loss, the best approach is to prevent damage and loss. The goals of therapy are more easily attained if a permanent loss does not have to be considered.

Hearing loss also affects language acquisition. Preschool cleft-palate children have been found to be significantly retarded in both receptive and expressive language (40). Awareness of the possibility of hearing loss and the importance of hearing health must be stressed. Preventive and restorative medicine helps eliminate or lessen hearing loss, but the best way to reduce middle-ear disease in the cleft-palate child over one year old is closure of the palate.

Those who deal with the cleft-palate individual must be aware of the possible presence of ear disease from birth. Conditions of hearing directly affect language development and speech quality.

Speech

Of the various deviations and deficiencies exhibited by individuals with clefts of the lip and palate, probably the most significant are those involving the process of speech communication. Although many discussions of the problem of speech deal primarily with the way the cleft-palate individual's speech sounds to the listener, there have also been investigations of the fundamental language structures. The language status of a cleft-palate child is important for both diagnostic information and treatment procedures.

There are some indications that, although cleft-palate children do experience a delay in all language areas, they tend to show improvement around the five-year age-level. Other studies indicate that these children retain their language retardation, and that the deficit even increases in significance as the child matures. This is not the same kind of speech retardation that the so-called delayed-speech child exhibits. Even though cleft-palate children may be intelligent and have large recognition vocabularies, they are still sometimes inhibited by their speech and by past experiences, which cause the retardation in mean sentence length and vocabulary usage. Morris (43) compared cleft-palate children with normal children and found that cleft-palate children were significantly retarded in their performance on the following language measures: (1) vocabulary, (2) mean sentence length, (3) structural complexity, (4) the number of different words used, and (5) articulation. He concluded that cleft-palate children have more than an anatomical defect. The indication here is that speech training must encompass more than articulation therapy or elimination of nasality. It must embody language teaching as well.

Defective articulation is, however, one of the major speech problems exhibited by individuals with clefts. It is generally agreed by present-day speech pathologists that the initial focus of direct speech therapy should be on the defects of articulation. Perhaps excessive attention has been given the problem of hypernasality in comparison to the correction of articulatory defects. It seems the wiser course of action to work first on correcting faulty articulation, since this adds measurably to speech intelligibility and since much of the hypernasality disappears as the oral movements and postures of syllable production are normalized.

The significance of nasality and nasal emission should not be minimized. Regardless of the language-proficiency level achieved or the percentage of errorless articulation, speech characterized by nasal emission or nasality is negatively distinguishing. The hypernasal sound of what is considered "typical" cleft-palate speech carries a prejudicial connotation; therefore, the elimination of nasal quality is certainly a major goal of therapy. It must be placed in proper perspective, however, and not emphasized to the exclusion of therapy aimed at making speech more intelligible. Of the two voice-quality problems—nasal emission and nasality—the former, because it is more distracting, is considered the more severe.

The chronology of therapeutic management appears to be: (1) the stimulation of language; (2) the correction of articulation defects; (3) the elimination of nasal quality. The areas are not separated into mutually exclusive segments of treatment since the therapies for each can be carried on simultaneously. The major focus of therapy management is in the order listed.

Chapter 6

A Final Word

Comments by Dr. Westlake at a Personal Interview

Around the time the senior author was completing his portion of this book, a friend of his, Dr. Harold Westlake, was participating in a symposium sponsored by the Educational Foundation of America Society of Plastic and Reconstructive Surgeons, which was being held at the Duke University Medical Center. Dr. Westlake was formerly Professor and Chairman of the Department of Communicative Disorders at Northwestern University and has had considerable experience working with cleft-palate patients and their families.

On May 1, 1973, in a personal interview with the senior author, Dr. Westlake was asked to discuss and define: (1) glottal stops, (2) pharyngeal fricatives, (3) nasality, (4) denasality, and (5) nasal emission. Though these terms have already been defined in this book, it will be to the advantage of the student to review how Dr. Westlake discussed and defined them on the basis of his years of experience in the profession of speech pathology. Dr. Westlake's definitions follow:

Glottal Stops: Many of the sounds we use in speaking are made by stopping off air or sound, and then releasing it quickly. For the /p/ we close the lips, damming up the air behind them, and then open them quickly. All there is to the /p/ sound is the noise that the puff of escaping air makes. We make a /t/ by stopping the air with the tip of the tongue, and then lowering the tongue quickly so the air rushes out. The /t/ we hear is simply the quick explosion of air released by the tongue tip.

Such sounds as /t/, /d/, /p/, /b/, /k/, and /g/ are all made by stopping air or sound and then letting it go quickly. We stop up the lips for /p/ and /b/; we stop air and sound at the tip of the tongue for /t/ and /d/; we close off the back of the mouth with the back of the tongue for /k/ and /g/. All of these sounds are called *stop* sounds.

A child with a cleft palate has a difficult job. He must learn our way of talking, but his mouth is different. He tries to make the sounds he hears other people use, but he cannot make them in the same way. When he tries to stop air with the tongue or lips, it rushes out through his nose. The only place where he can stop the air or sound is deep in the throat, at his larynx. This seems to be why almost all cleft-palate children will use a click, deep in the throat, for any stop consonant. This deep throat sound is called the *glottal stop*. It is a child's best way of making the stop sounds others make.

Pharyngeal Fricatives: Some sounds are made by forcing air and sound through narrow openings. For the /f/, we tighten the lips and drive the air through a small, tight opening between the lips. The friction or hissing of the escaping air is what we hear as the /f/. When we make an /s/, /sh/, /th/, or /z/, we force the air or sound through a small opening at the tip of the tongue. For these sounds, the sides and tip of the tongue press tightly against the teeth and gums, so the air cannot escape there. But at the center of the tip of the tongue, the tongue is pulled down just a little, so there is a very small opening to let the air and sound escape. The escaping air and sound can be recognized as an /s/, /th/, /sh/, etc., the particular sound heard depending only on the size of the hole. The smallest opening is for the /s/. The largest opening is for the /th/. The other sounds have openings that are in between the sizes required for the /s/ and /th/; but each one requires an opening of a definite size. Since each of these sounds results from the friction or hissing of air as it is forced through small openings of different sizes, they are called *fricative* sounds.

When the cleft-palate child tries to control air or sound with his lips or tongue, it escapes through the nose, so he is not successful. The only way he can use his tongue to control a small stream of air is to work farther back in his throat, behind the defective palate. So he fits his tongue against the back wall of his throat, and pushes the air through a small opening he leaves at the center of the back of the tongue. The throat is called the *pharynx*, so the fricative he makes is called a *pharyngeal fricative*. He can be expected to use this pharyngeal fricative for all of the fricative sounds others make with the lips and the front of the tongue. With his "different" speaking machine, this is his best way.

Nasality: The speech of many cleft-palate persons is often described as being *nasal*, or having *nasality*. In normal speech, the soft palate is lowered during the /m/, /n/, and /ng/ sounds, so these sounds come out through the nose. These three sounds are the only nasal sounds in normal speech. The soft palate is raised during all other English sounds, so none of the sound can get into the nose, and all of these sounds come out through the mouth.

A child with a cleft palate may have too short a palate, or the palate might not work well, so he cannot close off the opening to the nose that is at the back of the throat. When he tries to make the sounds that should come through the mouth, some sound will escape through the nose, and the speech has a "different" quality.

In saying the word *bay*, the soft palate should be raised or closed, and no sound should come through the nose. But in saying the word *may*, sound should come through the nose during the /m/, but none should come through the nose during the rest of the word, or the /ay/ part. When sound does come through the nose in words or parts of words that should have no nasal sound, the voices are said to be *nasal*. The problem is not just that the speaker sounds different, but since using nasal sound at the wrong times muffles the sounds that should come only through the mouth, the speaker is harder to understand.

Denasality: When a person's nose is blocked, or almost blocked, sound cannot come through the nose, even when it should. Such a person cannot make the sounds /m/, /n/, or /ng/, and he is said to be *denasal*. The denasal person's speech is not different just because those three nasal sounds are not heard. The denasal person usually tries so hard to make the nasal sounds that are difficult or impossible for him that he distorts the other sounds he should have no trouble in making.

A normal person can be denasal when the nose is congested with a cold or when the adenoid is large. Cleft-palate children may be denasal for a while after surgery on the palate. It is interesting that the average listener will usually say that denasal speech is worse than speech that has quite a bit of nasality.

Nasal Emission: What was written above about nasality helps us to understand *nasal emission*. When the palate does not work well, sound and air leak through the nose, even when a person is trying hard to direct all of the sound through the mouth. How much air or sound comes through the nose at the wrong time depends upon the sound the person is trying to make.

Sounds can be grouped in pairs, as /t-d/, /s-z/, /k-g/, etc. In each of these pairs the movement of the tongue in making them is exactly the same. The differences between the sounds in each pair are that the first sound in each pair is whispered and the second sound in each pair is voiced. In the voiced sounds, both air and sound will leak through the nose. In the whispered sounds, only air will leak through the nose. But we must remember that the whispered sounds are harder to hear, and so a person uses more effort in making them than he does making the voiced sounds. The result is that more air is emitted through the nose during whispered sounds than during voiced sounds.

When the air that comes through the nose during the whispered sounds can be heard, it is called a *nasal snort* or a *nasal emission*. And with many cleft-palate children, this nasal emission becomes very noticeable. It seems as if they are trying very hard to talk just like everyone else, and when they do not succeed with particular sounds, the natural result is for them to try even harder. Unfortunately, the harder they try, the worse they sound. The nasal emission becomes more and more noticeable.

Sometimes one sees a cleft-palate child having marked nasal snorts in his speech when they are not necessary. It may be that he learned to use a nasal snort at an early age, before he had surgery or a speech appliance. The habit of using a nasal snort for the correct sound can become so well established that he will continue to use it with a vengeance long after he might have been able to make correct sound.

Dr. Westlake also offered the following comments on two important matters:

Major mistakes parents make when they attempt to help their cleft-palate children speak better.

Parents of cleft-palate children are human beings; as such they are all different, and probably no two of them will make the same error. Possibly, instead of trying to anticipate a thousand different errors, one might try to list a few good things they can do:

1. When a child tries to talk, and his palate does not work properly, he seems instinctively to try to talk with the part of his speech machine that is behind the palate. This may be why he uses the glottal stops and pharyngeal fricatives described above in place of the sounds that are made with the lips or in the front of the mouth. We must remember that when the cleft-palate child is still very young, he must make decisions as to the best way for him to use his mechanism to make sounds. At an early age he often does not choose the best way. In emphasizing the back of the mechanism he makes a wrong decision.

Even very young children who are playing with sounds before they actually attempt to do real talking can be encouraged to use the lips and front of the tongue. Although these sounds will not be perfect, they are usually better and understood more easily than sounds made back in the throat. So, one good thing to do is to encourage them from the very beginning to "make sounds at the front of the mouth."

2. Encouraging a child to make sounds when his mouth and palate are not normal might seem like demanding the impossible. But usually it is not. Even when the palate is open, children can often make pretty good approximations of sounds if they make them very quietly. As early as seven or eight months children will mimic sounds, if it is done incidentally to playing or cuddling. If the parent makes the sounds very softly, the youngster will usually respond at the same low level.

Making sounds loudly and with force exaggerates the nasal escape of sound and air. In quieter production, this is not so noticeable.

3. In their efforts to help children talk, parents are likely to begin with particular sounds that are hard even for normal children to make. Sometimes they even try to get a two- or three-year-old to make good /s/ sounds. Normal children do not make this sound correctly before they are seven.

Generally, it is wise to start with the simplest sounds, and on the sounds a cleft-palate child may be expected to make successfully. They can usually make quite good vowel sounds. The nasal sounds, of course, are possible. The /p/, /b/, /t/, /d/, /l/, /k/, and /g/ can usually be made well enough to be recognized if made quietly. The /s/, /ch/, /z/, /sh/, and /th/ might well be left until later.

4. Rather than emphasizing the incorrect sounds in words, it is better to emphasize the good sounds in words. As was stated above, when a child tries very hard to make a sound that is difficult for him, he will distort other sounds in the word. Trying too hard with the one impossible sound interferes with his saying other sounds in a word that he can say. Pass over the difficult sounds, giving them less emphasis rather than stressing them. After all, a person is understood on the basis of words and sounds that he can say correctly, and not on the basis of words and sounds that he cannot make.

5. Careful study of cleft-palate speech has shown that these children learn in time to speak well enough to be understood but that they progress more slowly than the normals. The normal child shows little improvement after four or five years. He has mastered practically all of the English sounds by that time. However, the cleft-palate child can be expected to continue to improve up to as late as ten or twelve years. It seems in a way, that they have an awkward "talking machine," and it takes them longer to learn how to get the most from it. The lesson for the parents is that they can expect slow progress. The important thing is to keep on trying to help them and encourage them.

However, the study of cleft-palate speech is encouraging in that it seems that practically every cleft-palate child eventually gets speech that is readily understandable. But it takes time, much more than for the average child.

6. In the preschool years a large number of cleft-palate children have speech that is difficult to understand. Not being understood can be very discouraging for a child. Even though a parent will spend some time helping a child talk, there must be "free time" when the child is not stopped and asked to try to say a word better, or even asked what he said. Every child must enjoy talking, and when he is made to feel unsuccessful he will avoid talking. At times a parent will do well even to pretend that he understands.

Common errors made by speech therapists when they work with cleft-palate children. (It should be borne in mind that therapists are also human, and can make all of the errors a parent makes.)

There are many areas in speech correction that might be thought of as specialties. These would include aphasia, learning disorders, cerebral palsy, etc. The usual speech therapist might be thought of as a "general practitioner," one who can work well with the more common problems but who may not have had time to develop real expertise in special areas. Sometimes it is hard for the young therapist to admit he needs help, but it should be no more embarrassing than it would be for a dentist, a doctor, or a lawyer. Consultation is necessary in all fields.

The therapist's obligation is to arrange the best possible service for clients. If he is unsure of himself with a particular client, he should seek help. The best source of help would probably be from a university speech center, but even then care should be taken that the consultant has good knowledge of the cleft-palate problem. All university people do not.

Every cleft-palate child ought to be entitled to a speech evaluation by a person who is competent with this problem. The usual speech therapist can do a very good job with the training as outlined by the expert. Also, the therapist can work with more confidence. He cannot feel quite comfortable in the therapy situation when he is not sure of himself.

Additional Suggestions to Students

Besides reading additional books and studies dealing with speech and cleft palate, the student may want to investigate some of the many symposiums, short courses, and association meetings held annually. Such conferences offer much to both the beginning student and the experienced speech pathologist. Research and experimentation result in new knowledge, new methods, new devices, and modifications of older techniques, as well as confirmation of the appropriateness of many of the procedures which have been used for years. At the annual meeting of the American Cleft Palate Association, professionals from the various areas represented on the cleft-palate team come together for the presentation of research, the sharing of knowledge in the represented fields, and discussion of unresolved questions. Other organizations that have important conferences are the American Society of Plastic and Reconstructive Surgeons and the International Association of Logopedics and Phonitrics. Conferences, such as the Duke University Symposium on Oral-Facial Anomalies as Related to Speech Disorders, held annually, offer valuable experiences to persons interested in speech and cleft palate.

In addition to the annually scheduled meetings, there are many special conferences, short courses, and lectures held periodically throughout the nation. Many of these are in connection with university programs, medical centers, and rehabilitation organizations. Information concerning attendance may be obtained through college or university programs, rehabilitation centers, professional organizations, and publicity through the news media. Students' professional affiliation with the American Speech and Hearing Association and with their state speech and hearing association should serve as the most significant vehicle for their keeping informed regarding such conferences.

In addition to attending meetings, the student may want to view films such as the following teaching and research films produced by the senior author. The titles of these films are as follows:

1. *Rotational Cinefluorography*
2. *Characteristics of the Human Speech Mechanism as Studied by Cinefluorography*
3. *Different Aspects of Oral-Facial Anomalies as Related to Speech Disorders*
4. *The Duke Summer Speech Camp*

Other films which may be helpful are:

1. *Speakers with Cleft Palates*
2. *The Wisconsin Cleft Palate Story*

Conclusion

It is hoped that this introduction to the problem of cleft lip and palate will stimulate the reader to investigate the topic further, but even more that it can serve to indicate the validity of McDonald's assertion:

Yes, with professional help from the specialists and understanding guidance from his parents, the child born with a cleft lip or a cleft palate has a bright future (18).

Appendix

Specific Therapeutic Techniques Used in Cleft-Palate Habilitation

In considering techniques it must be remembered that techniques are important but have no value when used mechanically. A listing of techniques, then, is for the purpose of reference. The therapeutic process is characterized by continued diagnosis. Inherent in this is the choice, use, and evaluation of techniques. Some, which appear to hold the promise of usefulness, will prove ineffective; others, lacking appeal, may prove useful. The following suggestions are just that—suggestions. The actual list of techniques is limited only by the therapist's imagination and creativity.

I. TONGUE EXERCISES

A. Create awareness of tongue position and place of contact.
   1. Therapist touches spots on tongue, lips, and in the mouth and pharynx, and client touches exact same points (use a swab stick).
   2. Therapist touches two points of contact which client should make for specific sounds.
   3. Therapist has client raise dorsum of tongue around bowl of spoon.
B. Exercises to increase tongue mobility.
   1. Therapist tells story for "Sweep the house" or "Paint the fence" while client does the movements with tongue to represent the story.
   2. Follow movements of objects with tongue (airplane, car, flag, bird, etc.).
   3. Therapist has client follow movements on count, as "on count of one stick out your tongue, on count of two, pull it back in, on count of three close lips." Count "one, two, three." Other exercises include pointing tongue, grooving tongue, lateralizing tongue, etc.
   4. Rapid protrusion and retraction of tongue.
   5. Sing "London Bridge Is Falling Down" using la, la, la instead of the words.
   6. Put peanut butter on palate at y position. Have client use dorsum of tongue to remove peanut butter.
   7. Use exercises from tongue-thrust assignments.

II. LIP EXERCISES FOR TIGHT AND INERT UPPER LIP

1. Imitation of pictures illustrating exaggerated lip positions for vowels.
2. Play "Simon Says" with therapist making exaggerated faces (smiling, frowning, wide mouth openings, pouting lips, etc.). Client imitates with both therapist and client looking in mirror.
3. Rapid protrusion and retraction of lip musculature.
4. Raising the upper lip to display the gum ridge.
5. Successive retraction of the right and the left sides of the mouth.
6. Opening and closing of the lips in a protruded position.
7. If lower lip protrudes, adapt above exercises. Stimulate approximation of the lips for longer periods of time.

III. EXERCISES TO ESTABLISH ARTICULATORY PLACEMENT OF SOUNDS

1. Fish talk—*p* and *m* sounds—a clicking sound which results when relaxed, moistened lips are tapped together lightly as the mandible is elevated and lowered.
2. Establish larger mouth opening. Begin with open vowels.
3. Emphasize light contacts in making *t* and *d* sounds. Depress mandible and tap the gum ridge with tongue tip. Do same for *n*, *l*, and *r*.
4. Practice plosive consonants with the following: hum, occlude nostrils, produce *p* and *b*.
5. Practice *s* and *z* sounds with light closure between teeth and stress correct placement; use short oral air flow; make *s* by going from *t* to *s*, from *th* to *s*, and from *f* to *s*.
6. Practice *k* and *g* by holding tongue tip down as client tries to produce *t* sound.
7. Since final consonants are often easier to produce, practice *ahp—ah*, *ahp—ah*, *ahp—ay*, *ahp—ee*.
8. For syllable drill, begin with *ah*. This is usually easiest for the cleft-palate individual since the soft palate is not raised quite so high as it is for *oo* and *ee*, and there is less resistance to the passage of air through the mouth, the tongue being flat.
9. For word and sentence drill, use general carry-over methods employed in any articulation therapy.

IV. EAR TRAINING EXERCISES

A. Practice auditory discrimination between nasal and nonnasal word pairs, nasal and nonnasal paragraphs (these can be found in most voice and diction drill books).

B. Client must recognize own voice quality. Tape-recordings may be a shock, but client must hear his voice quality if he is to reduce it. His procedure would include:
  1. Accepting the recording.
  2. Analyzing it.
  3. Varying his voice quality.
  4. Reducing nasality.

V. PROCEDURES FOR VOICE THERAPY

  A. Exercises to reduce nasal tone and to improve resonance.
     1. Practice relaxation of tongue on the floor of the mouth.
     2. Practice vowel *ah* with tongue flat and relaxed. Also *oo* and *ee*.
     3. Emphasize open mouth; do not permit closed teeth during practice; do not permit tip of tongue in mouth opening during practice.
     4. Hum *m* or *n*, closing one nostril at a time, then with both open.
     5. Hum, gradually open mouth on vowel sound.
     6. Begin whistling and gradually add humming, until whistling and humming at the same time.
     7. Work from vowel which is less nasalized than others.
  B. Compensatory therapy.
     1. Practice wider mouth opening.
     2. Contrast voice with more then less force.

VI. EXERCISES FOR DEVELOPING CORRECT BREATH DIRECTION AND THE USE OF THE PALATOPHARYNGEAL SPHINCTER

     1. Whistling.
     2. Playing wind instruments.
     3. Playing suction games.
     4. Humming.
     5. Yawning.
        a. Breathe in on a yawn position and out on a vowel shape without a sound.
        b. Breathe in on a yawn position and out on a voiced vowel.
        c. Think the yawn position; voice a sound—use a mirror.
     6. Practice conscious movement of the soft palate (repeat *ah* while observing in mirror).
     7. Use alternation of vowel and nasal resonance, e.g., *ah—ng*.
     8. Practice holding air under pressure in the mouth.
        a. Blow out cheek, holding nostrils if necessary.
        b. Blow down nose, interrupt air pressure by raising palate and closing sphincter.
        c. Alternate oral and nasal emission of air.

VII. EXERCISES FOR COORDINATION OF THE PALATOPHARYNGEAL SPHINCTER AND MUSCLES OF ARTICULATION

(Begin with one consonant, *p* is generally easiest.)

1. Hold air under pressure in the mouth and release it through the palatopharyngeal sphincter, keeping the lips closed.
2. Hum (the sphincter being slightly open), then deflect the breath into the mouth, distending the cheeks (sphincter closed).
3. Hum—blow out cheeks—hum, alternately.
4. Hum—blow out cheeks—release on *p*.
5. Blow out cheeks—relax lips—articulate *p* (occlude nares).
6. Alternately open and close the sphincter rapidly as in *m—pah, m—pay, m—po, m—poo*.
7. Practice the above more rapidly to approximate speech required in normal speech. Also use *n* and *ng* in this exercise.
8. Omit the nasal sound and practice using the plosive consonant alone in *pah, pay, pee, po, poo* and *pah, pah, pah*; *pay, pay, pay*; etc.
9. Practice using *p* as a final sound as in *ahp*.

VIII. TREATMENT TO OVERCOME THE USE OF THE GLOTTAL STOP

1. Use easy but careful production of all sounds.
2. Humming—start with a slight puff of air down the nose, let the client hum gently, then add vowels.
3. Whispering—breathe in and out easily through the mouth for relaxation. Begin with easy vowels, then voiceless consonants, then voiced consonants.
4. Close anterior nares to prevent nasal escape.
5. Therapist may begin plosive articulation by moving client's lower lip with his (therapist's) fingers sufficiently to allow the release of air.

IX. TREATMENT FOR PHARYNGEAL OR LARYNGEAL FRICATIVES

1. Breathe in, occlude nostrils, blow gently through almost closed lips, change teeth and lower lip to *f* and continue. Repeat.
2. Go from correctly produced fricative to another, from *f—s*.
3. Have patient whistle and go from that to target sound.

X. DEVELOPMENT OF CONTROL OF FACIAL EXPRESSION

1. Use mirror or videotape to practice articulation. Observe facial expression.
2. Use mirror or videotape to alter facial expressions.
3. Use hands or fingers to prevent undesirable facial movements.

XI. SENSORY STIMULATION

1. Stroke tissues to increase tactile sensation.
2. Apply pressure or have client tighten muscles around an object to increase resistance.
3. Use chilled, warmed, or roughened objects for stimulation.
4. The speech bulb on a temporary appliance provides both tactile stimulation and resistance.

References

1. P. P. Phillips. "Author's Guide," Cliffs Speech and hearing series. Auburn, Ala., 1972.
2. E. Pickrell. Cleft lip and associated problems. Paper presented at the Third Annual Duke University Symposium on Orofacial Anomalies as Related to Speech Disorders, Durham, N.C., 1971.
3. P. Fogh-Andersen. Recent statistics of facial clefts frequency, heredity, mortality. In R. Hotz (ed.), *Early treatment of cleft lip and palate—International Symposium April 9–11, 1964.* University of Zurich, Dental Institute. Berne and Stuttgart: Hans Huber Publishers, 1964.
4. W. H. Olin. *Cleft Lip and Palate Rehabilitation.* Springfield, Ill.: Charles C. Thomas, 1960.
5. W. Zemlin. *Speech and Hearing Science Anatomy and Physiology.* Champaign, Ill.: Stipes Publishing Co., 1964.
6. H. Lane. Drugs known to induce cleft palate and/or cleft lip in experimental animals. In *An integrated program concerned with habilitation-rehabilitation of oral-facial-communicative disorders.* Lancaster, Pa.: Lancaster Cleft Palate Clinic, 1966.
7. J. Warkany and E. Schraffenberger. Congenital malformations induced in rats by maternal nutritional deficiency. V. Effects of a purified diet lacking riboflavin. *Proc. Soc. Exp. Biol. Med.,* 1943, 54:92–94.
8. F. M. Deuschle, J. F. Geiger, and J. Warkany. Analysis of an anomalous oculodentofacial pattern in newborn rats produced by maternal hypervitaminosis. *Amer. J. Dent. Res.,* 1959, 38:149–55.
9. F. C. Fraser, T. D. Fainstat, and H. Kalter. *Etudes Neo-Natales,* 1953, 2, 43.
10. J. Warkany, P. H. Beaudry, and S. Hornstein. Attempted abortion with 4-amino-pteroylglutamic acid (aminopterin); malformations of the child. *Amer. J. Dis. Child.,* 1959, 97, 274–81. (Also in *Obstet. Gynec. Survey,* 1960, 15, 1.)
11. J. Longacre. *Cleft Palate Deformation.* Springfield, Ill.: Charles C. Thomas, 1970.
12. C. Van Riper and J. V. Irwin. *Voice and articulation.* Englewood Cliffs, N.J.: Prentice-Hall, 1964.
13. G. Snyder, S. Berkowitz, K. Bzoch, and S. Stool. *Your Cleft Lip and Palate Child: A Basic Guide for Parents.* Florida Cleft Palate Association and Mead Johnson Laboratories.

14. K. Pickrell, N. Georgiade, F. Morris, and J. Adamson. Plastic surgical conditions in infancy and childhood. *Postgrad. Med.*, 1960, 27, 705.
15. R. Massengill. *Hypernasality: Considerations in Causes and Treatment Procedures.* Springfield, Ill.: Charles C. Thomas, 1972.
16. M. E. Morley. *Cleft Palate and Speech.* Baltimore: Williams & Wilkins, 1966.
17. C. Van Riper. *Speech Correction: Principles and Methods.* (3rd ed.). Englewood Cliffs, N.J.: Prentice-Hall, 1954.
18. E. T. McDonald. *Bright promise.* Chicago: National Easter Seal Society for Crippled Children and Adults, 1959.
19. H. Westlake and D. Rutherford. *Cleft Palate.* Englewood Cliffs, N.J.: Prentice-Hall, 1966.
20. W. Grabb, S. Rosenstein, and K. Bzoch (eds.). *Cleft Lip and Palate: Surgical, Dental, and Speech Aspects.* Boston: Little, Brown, 1971.
21. N. Georgiade, E. Clifford, and R. Massengill. *The Child with Cleft Lip or Palate: A Guide for Parents.* A publication made possible by a grant from The National Foundation-March of Dimes, 1973.
22. J. Eisenson and M. Ogilvie. *Speech Correction in the Schools.* New York: Macmillan, 1967.
23. Travis, L. E. (ed.). *Handbook of Speech Pathology and Audiology.* New York: Appleton-Century-Crofts, 1971.
24. H. Morris. The oral manometer as a diagnostic tool in clinical speech pathology. *J. Speech & Hearing Dis.*, 1966, 31, 362–69.
25. C. Van Riper. *Speech Correction: Principles and Methods.* (4th ed.). Englewood Cliffs, N.J.: Prentice-Hall, 1964.
26. R. Massengill, G. Quinn, K. Pickrell, and C. Levinson. Therapeutic exercise and velopharyngeal gap. *Cleft Palate J.*, 1968, 5, 44–47.
27. R. Massengill, G. Quinn, and K. Pickrell. The use of a palatal stimulator to decrease velopharyngeal gap. *Ann. Otol., Rhinol., & Laryngol.*, 1971, 80, 135.
28. A. C. Roberts. *Obturators and Prostheses for Cleft Palate: Their Use and Construction.* London: E. & S. Livingstone, 1965.
29. O. E. Beder. *Surgical and Maxillofacial Prosthesis.* Seattle: University of Washington Press, 1959.
30. R. Yules. *Atlas for Surgical Repair of Cleft Lip-Cleft Palate and Non-Cleft Velopharyngeal Incompetence.* Springfield, Ill.: Charles C. Thomas, 1971.
31. J. Converse. *Reconstructive Plastic Surgery.* Vol. 3. Philadelphia: W. B. Saunders, 1968.
32. B. McWilliams. Some factors in the intelligibility of cleft palate speech. *J. Speech & Hearing Dis.*, 1954, 19, 524–27.
33. C. S. Harkins and H. K. Baker. Twenty-five years of cleft palate prosthesis. *J. Speech & Hearing Dis.*, 1948, 13, 23–30.
34. M. Berry and J. Eisenson. *Speech Disorders: Principles and Practices of Therapy.* New York: Appleton-Century Crofts, 1956.
35. E. Clifford. Cleft palate and the person: Psychologic studies of its impact. *S. Med. J.*, 1971, 64, 1516–20.
36. J. Kallaus. The child with cleft lip and palate. *Amer. J. Nursing*, 1965, 65, 120–23.

37. K. R. Bzoch (ed.). *Communicative Disorders Related to Cleft Lip and Palate.* Boston: Little, Brown, 1972.
38. V. Tisza and E. Gumpertz. The parents' reaction to the birth and early care of children with cleft palate. *Pediatrics,* 1962, 30, 86–90.
39. E. Crocker and C. Crocker. Some implications of superstitions and folk beliefs for counseling parents of children with cleft lip and cleft palate. *Cleft Palate J.,* 1970, 7, 124–28.
40. R. Yules. Hearing in cleft palate patients. *Arch. Otolaryngol.,* 1970, 91, 319–23.
41. H. Davis and S. R. Silverman. *Hearing and Deafness.* New York: Holt, Rinehart & Winston, 1960.
42. R. Harrison. Observations on hearing of preschool cleft palate children. *J. Speech & Hearing Dis.,* 1971, 36, 252–56.
43. H. Morris. Communication skills of children with cleft palate and cleft lip. *J. Speech & Hearing Res.,* 1962, 5, 79–90.
44. R. B. Yules. Secondary correction of velopharyngeal incompetence: a review. *Plastic and Reconstructive Surgery,* 1970, 45, 234–46.

Glossary of Technical Terms

Words set in SMALL CAPS are defined elsewhere in the Glossary

Adenoids
Enlargement of the lymphoid tissue on the posterior wall of the nasopharynx.

Alveolar
Pertaining to the ridges on the MANDIBLE and MAXILLA that overlie the roots of the teeth.

Articulation
The movements of the speech organs during speech to modify the voiced and unvoiced breath stream to form meaningful sounds; the speech function performed by the tongue, lips, teeth, MANDIBLE, and soft palate or VELUM.

Assimilation
The modification of a speech sound by the influence of sounds of adjacent sounds or sounds made in close proximity.

Audiologist
Specialist in the science of hearing.

Audiology
The study of hearing and hearing disorders.

Bifid
Divided into two parts; cleft, as a bifid UVULA.

Bilateral
Related to two sides; pertaining to or affecting both sides.

Blade
The flattened upper and forward portion of the tongue, which is capable of distension and extension.

Cinefluorography
X-ray motion pictures.

Cleft lip
A congenital cleft of the upper lip, usually on one side only, sometimes on both sides, but rarely medially; sometimes extending into the nostrils, but may be so slight as to be only a notch in the upper lip. Also called *chiloschisis* and *harelip*.

Cleft palate

A congenital cleft of the roof of the mouth, involving the soft palate only or the soft palate and hard palate, and sometimes extending through the ALVEOLAR ridge and into the lip (where it is called cleft lip); can occur on either or both sides. Also called *uranoschisis*.

Congenital

Existing at birth, either a hereditary condition or a pathology following conception of the embryo (always refers to a disease, deformity, or deficiency).

Consonant

A speech sound, voiced or voiceless, the chief characteristic of which is a nonmusical friction noise generated by driving the expired air through so narrow an opening as to raise its pressure and thus its speech, so as to convert sounds that have been ascribed meaning in a language.

Cosmetic

Pertaining to beautification, as in cosmetic surgery, which is performed for the purpose of making a person more attractive.

Dental

Pertaining to the teeth.

Dorsum

The back; the superior surface of the tongue.

Etiology

The cause of an abnormal condition; the study of such cause.

Eustachian

Relating to the tube or passageway connecting the PHARYNX with the middle ear.

Fricative

Any speech sound made by forcing the air stream through such a narrow opening that audible high-frequency sounds are made, such as *th*, *f*, *s*.

Glottal stop

A plosive sound made by impounding the air stream beneath the closed GLOTTIS and then suddenly releasing it; sometimes called *glottal click*; phonetically represented /ʔ/.

Glottis

The open space between the vocal folds when they are not approximated.

Guttural

Pertaining to the throat, as a guttural sound meaning a sound made in the throat, or throaty.

Hard-of-hearing

Having reduced hearing acuity; any degree of lessened auditory acuity short of complete deafness.

Harelip
> *See* CLEFT LIP.

Hearing loss
> The amount of impairment of a person's hearing measured in terms of comparison with normal hearing ability.

Hyper-
> A prefix designating a greater amount or degree, as *hypernasality* (too much nasality).

Hypo-
> A prefix designating a lesser amount or degree, as *hyponasality* (too little nasality).

Laryngology
> The medical science concerned with systematized knowledge of the LARYNX; pathology of the larynx.

Larynx
> The voice box; that portion of the respiratory mechanism containing the vocal folds.

Malocclusion
> A failure of the teeth of the lower jaw to meet those of the upper jaw properly.

Mandible
> The lower jaw.

Manometer
> An instrument used for measuring the pressure of liquids or gases, as for measuring nasal air pressure in cleft-palate individuals.

Maxilla
> The upper jaw. The part of the skeleton of the head that forms the roof of the mouth, the floor of the nasal cavity, and the mounting of the upper teeth. (Strictly speaking, it does not include that portion of the palatal bone that mounts the incisors. That portion is the PREMAXILLA.)

Maxillofacial
> Pertaining to the lower half of the face and to a subdivision of surgery dealing with this area of the face.

Molar
> Any of the three permanent, or two deciduous, back teeth on each side of each jaw.

Nasal
> Pertaining to the nose or to the nasal cavities; with reference to speech sounds, any sound coming through the nose, giving it a distinctive resonant quality referred to as nasal.

Nasal cavity

The passageway from outer air to the PHARYNX; the right and left nasal cavities are separated by the nasal SEPTUM.

Nasal port

The passageway from the oral cavity to the NASAL CAVITY separated by the action of the soft palate (velum) and the superior pharyngeal constrictor.

Nasality

Having nasal quality.

Nasopharyngeal occlusion

See PALATOPHARYNGEAL CLOSURE.

Nasopharynx

The upper part of the PHARYNX, continuous with the nasal passages.

Obturator

Any structure that closes an opening, especially an artificial plate to close a cleft in the palate.

Organic

Referring to organs of the body, as an organic cause as opposed to a functional cause.

Orthodontics

The branch of dentistry concerned with the treatment of MALOCCLUSION.

Otolaryngologist

A physician skilled in the practice of OTOLOGY, RHINOLOGY, and LARYNGOLOGY.

Otology

The medical science concerned with the diagnosis and treatment of individuals who have an ear disease or disorders of the peripheral mechanism of hearing.

Palatal stimulator

A palatal stimulator, or lift, is an oral appliance that usually covers part of the hard palate and has an extension that fits against the soft palate and may help raise up the soft palate.

Palate

The roof of the mouth, including the anterior portion (the hard palate) and the posterior portion (the soft palate, or velum).

Palatopharyngeal closure

Separation of nasal and oral cavities by effecting a seal with the posterior third portion of the soft palate raised against the pharyngeal wall.

Passavant's pad

A bulging on the posterior pharyngeal wall. Also called *Passavant's cushion* and *Passavant's bar.*

Pharynx
The throat; the part of the respiratory tract that extends from the NASAL CAVITY to the larynx; for purposes of site identification may be divided into three parts: (1) the nasopharynx, the portion immediately posterior to the NASAL CAVITY; (2) the oropharynx, the portion immediately posterior to the oral cavity; and (3) the laryngopharynx, the portion immediately above the larynx.

Phonate
To produce voice by means of vibration of the vocal folds.

Plastic surgery
A specialized branch of surgery concerned with building up tissues, restoring lost parts, repairing or rectifying malformations or defects.

Plosive
Any speech sound made by impounding the air stream for a moment, until considerable pressure has been developed, and then suddenly releasing it, as in *p, d.*

Posterior
Pertaining to, located in, or directed toward the back part of the body, the back part of an organ. Opposite: *anterior.*

Premaxilla
The portion of the upper jaw bone upon which are mounted the four incisors.

Prenatal
Pertaining to the conditions of life of the embryo and fetus; condition before birth.

Postnatal
Pertaining to condition or event following birth.

Prosthesis
An artificial substitute for a missing part, as denture, hand, palate.

Prosthodontist
A dentist who specializes in prosthetic dentistry.

Resonance
Modification of the vocal sound by passage through the cavities of the throat and head so as to alter its quality.

Rhinology
The medical science concerned with the treating of the nose and its diseases.

Septum
The bony and cartilagineous partition separating the two principal NASAL CAVITIES.

Speech
The faculty of expressing thought by spoken words; the act of speaking; the spoken words.

Speech pathologist
A specialist in the science of speech and language disorders.

Sphincter
A muscle surrounding and closing an orifice, a mechanism for closing a passageway.

Submucous cleft
A cleft or opening in the submucuosa or layer of fibrous connective tissue that attaches the mucous membrane to its adjacent parts.

Uvula
The pendular tip or POSTERIOR termination of the VELUM.

Velopharyngeal closure
See PALATOPHARYNGEAL CLOSURE.

Velopharyngeal seal
See PALATOPHARYNGEAL CLOSURE.

Velopharyngeal sufficiency
See PALATOPHARYNGEAL CLOSURE.

Velum
The soft palate.

Bibliography

BEDER, O. *Surgical and Maxillofacial Prostheses*. Seattle: University of Washington Press, 1959. This little booklet provides basic information for those interested in surgical and maxillofacial prostheses.

BZOCH, K. R. (Ed.) *Communicative Disorders Related to Cleft Lip and Palate*. Boston: Little, Brown, 1972. This book is a comprehensive study of the condition of cleft lip and palate as they relate to speech and language. Offering contributions by twenty-four authors, it contains a great deal of research on the different topics discussed and covers many diverse aspects of the problem of cleft palate. It would be a very useful source book for speech-pathology students.

GEORGIADE, N., CLIFFORD, E., and MASSENGILL, R. *The Child with Cleft Lip or Palate: A Guide for Parents*. A publication made possible by a grant from the National Foundation–March of Dimes, 1973. This work is a guide for parents, helping them to understand the problem of cleft palate, its treatment, and the prognosis for habilitation. It could be useful in parent counseling.

HOTZ, R. (Ed.) *Early Treatment of Cleft Lip and Palate*. Berne, Hans Huber, 1964. This publication covers an international symposium conducted April 9–11, 1964. It provides a most useful review concerning aspects of orthodontic treatment as related to cleft palate.

LONGACRE, J. *Cleft Palate Deformation*. Springfield, Ill.: Charles C. Thomas, 1970. This book contains excellent materials dealing with the many facets of cleft-palate deformation. The pictorial presentations are clear and easy to follow.

McDONALD, E. T. *Bright Promise*. Chicago: National Easter Seal Society for Crippled Children and Adults, 1959. This small booklet, written for the parents of children with cleft lip and palate, explains causes, repair, and associated problems and indicates that such children have a bright future. It would be quite suitable for the parents of a cleft-palate infant.

MASSENGILL, R. *Hypernasality: Considerations in Causes and Treatment Procedures*. Springfield, Ill.: Charles C. Thomas, 1972. This book deals with the specific speech problem of hypernasality and presents a comprehensive analysis of the problem with suggested therapy procedures. It could be very useful to the student and therapist.

MORLEY, M. E. *Cleft Palate and Speech.* Baltimore: Williams & Wilkins, 1966. The author presents a very complete treatment of the problem of cleft palate, beginning with the growth of the embryo, tracing the historical development of surgical procedures, and giving suggestions for treatment. The date of its original publication was 1945, but the book has been so popular that seven editions have been printed since then.

RAHN, A. O., and BOUCHER, L. J. *Maxillofacial Prosthetics: Principles and Concepts.* Philadelphia: W. B. Saunders, 1970. This book covers the construction of all types of prosthetics, with one chapter devoted to cleft-palate prosthetics. It is written in language that the speech-pathology student can understand and would serve to aid the student in understanding the area of prosthetic appliances.

ROBERTS, A. C. *Obturators and Prostheses for Cleft Palate.* Edinburgh: E. & S. Livingston, 1965. This booklet, along with the one by Beder, provides pertinent information concerning the utilization and construction of oral prostheses used in cleft-palate habilitation.

SPRIESTERSBACH, D. C., and SHERMAN, D. (Eds.) *Cleft Palate and Communication.* New York: Academic Press, 1968. The editors present a very complete and detailed analysis of the speech problems associated with cleft palate, with contributions by ten different authorities in the field. This would be a good handbook for the speech-pathology student.

STARK, R. (Ed.) *Cleft Palate: A Multidiscipline Approach.* New York: Harper & Row, 1968. This book, with contributions by a number of authors, deals with the many aspects and specialities involved in cleft-palate treatment.

WESTLAKE, H., and RUTHERFORD, D. *Cleft Palate.* Englewood Cliffs, N.J.: Prentice-Hall, 1966. This book provides a very good synopsis of the speech problems encountered by the cleft-palate patient and the therapeutic procedures that may be involved.